AF885071

Managing Knee Arthritis at Home: A Physiotherapy Perspective

A Practical and Holistic Approach to Maximize Mobility and Improve the Quality of Life

Dr. Priya Reddappa, PT

Managing Knee Arthritis at Home: A Physiotherapy Perspective

Author: Dr. Priya Reddappa, PT

First Edition: 2025

Copyright © 2025 Priya Reddappa.

All rights reserved. No part of this publication may be reproduced or transmitted in any form or by any means, electronic, mechanical, photocopying, recording, any information storage or retrieval system or otherwise, without the prior permission in writing from the author. Please purchase only authorized electronic or print editions and do not participate or encourage in the electronic piracy of the copyrighted material.

ISBN: 978-93-342-6685-6

Published by: Priya Reddappa

DISCLAIMER

The information provided in this book is for educational purposes only and is based on the author's experience and research. This book is not intended to make any diagnosis or provide treatment for any medical condition. Please consult your primary care physician and therapist before beginning any exercise or treatment provided in this book. The information in the book is to be followed or used after discussion with the therapist and under the therapist's care and supervision. The author and the publisher do not assume responsibility and are not liable to any party for any damages, loss, errors, injuries, or negative consequences resulting from reading or following the information provided in this book. The author and the publisher are not responsible for any health needs requiring medical supervision, an increase in symptoms, or any health problem resulting from using the information in this book.

With the blessings of Shri Shirdi Sai Baba,

this work has been possible.

I dedicate this book to my family,

whose love, support and encouragement

had been tremendous during the writing of this book.

ABOUT THE AUTHOR

Priya Reddappa, MPT (Paediatric Neurology), APGDCR-PV, is a postgraduate Paediatric Physical Therapist, and a licensed Life Member of Indian Association of Physiotherapists (MIAP). She completed her Masters in Physical Therapy (Paediatric Neurology) from The Tamil Nadu Dr M.G.R Medical University and has experience as a Physical Therapist over 12 years in various clinical areas of Orthopaedics, Neurology, Cardiorespiratory, and Neuropaediatric conditions. As a clinically driven professional, she has worked in paediatric acute care (inpatient settings), outpatient settings, special school, and paediatric rehabilitation centres. She has handled paediatric patients at Apollo Children's Hospital, Chennai for over five years. She gained experience as a Research Clinical Evaluator for Apollo Hospitals Education and Research Foundation for a Clinical Trial on Duchenne Muscular Dystrophy for about four years. She has published two research papers in international journals regarding hand function in children with cerebral palsy, and adults with spinal cord injury. She is focused on providing high quality, cost effective Physical Therapy services and implementing treatment programs in order to bring comfort, hope and wellness to her patients.

ACKNOWLEDGEMENT

I thank all the authors, whose books helped me derive my knowledge during my graduation and apply it into my clinical practice as a Physical Therapist. I also thank the authors listed in the references at the end of this book, whose work has helped me to use the information to guide the readers of this book to further their knowledge in managing knee pain issues.

Priya Reddappa

TABLE OF CONTENTS

UNDERSTANDING KNEE ARTHRITIS

THE ANATOMY OF THE KNEE JOINT

Understanding the anatomy and the functions of the knee joint is useful to prevent and treat injuries, as well as for maintaining the overall joint health.

The knee joint is a type of hinge joint (that allows movement in only one plane) connecting the thigh bone (femur) to the shin bone (tibia). The largest sesamoid bone, called the patella, is located at the anterior of the knee joint. Sesamoid bones commonly develop in tendons or muscles at a place where they cross the joints. Patella is called a sesamoid, and it is found within a muscle called the quadriceps. The joint also derives support from the fibula, which is a smaller bone located on the lateral (outer) side of the tibia. The knee joint is responsible for allowing movements such as flexion (knee bending), extension (knee straightening), and rotation.

Anatomy of the knee joint

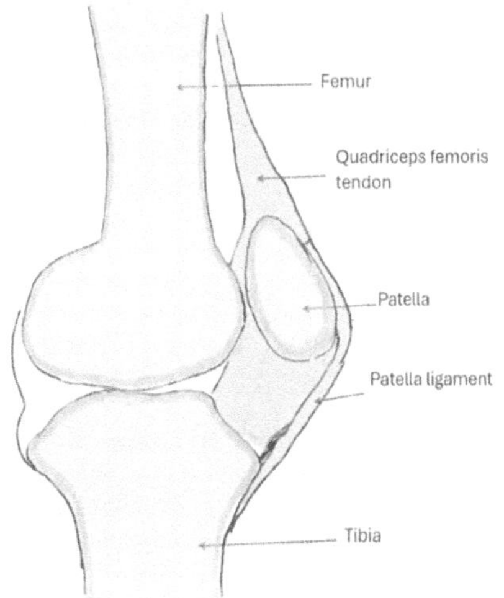

The knee joint is formed by the articulation of the femoral condyles and the tibial plateau. The femoral condyles, namely the medial and the lateral, are the rounded parts of the femur that form the knee joint, while the tibial plateau is the flat part of the tibia over which the femoral condyles rest on.

The knee joint complex consists of two joints: the joint between the femur and tibia called the tibiofemoral joint and the joint between the patella and femur called the patellofemoral joint.

The knee joint is held in place by several strong ligaments. The anterior cruciate ligament (ACL) and posterior cruciate ligament (PCL) run diagonally through the knee joint and help stabilise it. The ACL and PCL work together, thus preventing excessive forward or backward movement of the tibia on the thigh bone. The medial collateral ligament (MCL) and lateral collateral ligament (LCL) run along the sides of the joint and help prevent the knee from excessive bending and the side-to-side movement of the tibia on the femur.

Ligaments of the knee joint

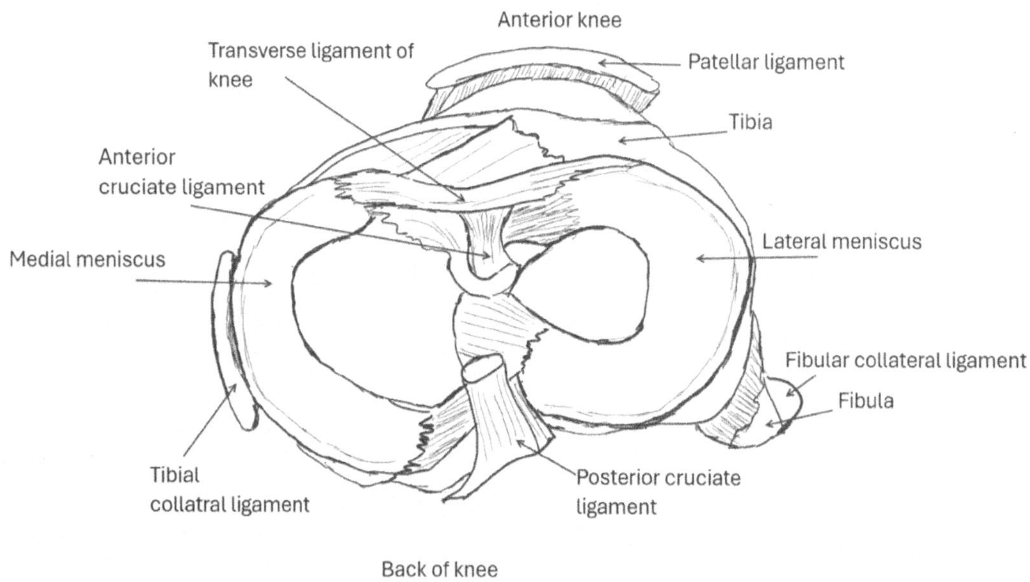

The knee joint also has two menisci, which are crescent-shaped pieces of cartilage. They help the knee joint as shock absorbers between the femur and tibia. The meniscus is made of fibrous cartilage and facilitates appropriate force distribution in the knee joint. The menisci also help to distribute weight evenly across the joint and provide stability. The meniscus acts as a cushion between the bones, absorbing shock and reducing the amount of stress on the joint.

The knee joint is also lined by a layer of smooth, glossy tissue called the synovial membrane, which produces synovial fluid to lubricate the joint and reduce friction. The synovial membrane also provides nutrition for the joint.

The knee joint is innervated by the femoral nerve, which provides sensation to the front of the thigh and knee, and the obturator nerve, which provides sensation to the medial aspect of the thigh and knee. The knee joint is also supplied by the femoral artery and the popliteal artery, which provide blood to the knee joint and surrounding muscles.

Injuries to the knee joint can occur as a result of a traumatic event or from overuse. Common injuries include ACL and MCL sprains, meniscus tears, and patellofemoral pain syndrome (PFPS).

BIOMECHANICS OF THE KNEE JOINT

The movements at the knee joint occur in three planes: the sagittal, coronal, and transverse planes. The movements of flexion and extension occur in the sagittal plane, while the medial and lateral rotation occur in the coronal plane.

- Flexion refers to the movement of decreasing the angle between the thigh and the leg, such as when sitting down or bending the knee
- Extension refers to the movement of increasing the angle between the thigh and the leg, such as when standing up or straightening the knee

Movements of the knee joint

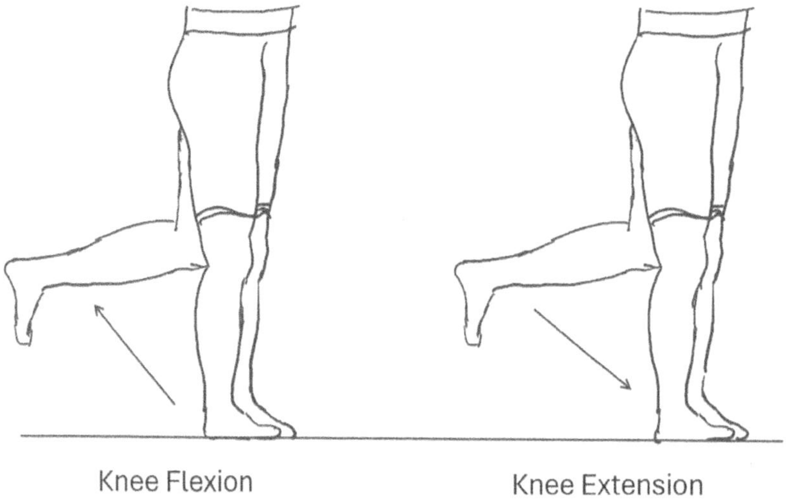

- Medial rotation refers to the movement of rotating the knee inward, towards the midline of the body
- Lateral rotation refers to the movement of rotating the knee outward, away from the midline of the body

- Some degree of circumduction involving flexion, extension, and medial and lateral rotation is also allowed. But as the knee joint is a type of hinge joint, the amount of circumduction and rotation is limited
- The knee also has a small amount of glide and slide in the coronal plane, which is called anteroposterior translation. Anterior translation refers to the movement of the knee sliding forward, and posterior translation refers to the movement of the knee sliding backward

The knee joint is a hinge joint, and as such, it does not allow for rotation in the transverse plane. The tibiofemoral joint aids in transmitting the body weight from the femur to the tibia and allows for some hinge-like rotation movements to occur in small degrees axially (Chhabra et al., 2001). During movements such as walking, running, or jumping, the knee joint works in coordination with the hip and ankle joints to create smooth and efficient movements.

SCREW HOME MECHANISM IN THE KNEE JOINT

A screw home mechanism is how the knee joint works to provide more stability when standing and walking. During the knee straightening, the femur rotates inwards on the tibia, and during knee bending, the femur rotates outwards. These movements of internal and external rotation of the femur are controlled by the ligaments, ACL and PCL, thus preventing excessive forward and backward movement of the tibia. This movement is important for walking and running. The shape of the femur's lower part (femoral condyles) and the shape of the upper part of the tibia (tibial plateau) are responsible for the screw home mechanism. Screw home mechanism occurs due to the difference in the size of the medial and lateral condyles of the femur and the difference in the surface areas that exist in the medial and lateral tibial plateaus.

The knee joint is coordinated well by the muscles, bones, ligaments, tendons, and bursae not only in complex knee movements but also in tolerating the tremendous forces exerted on it (Zhang et al., 2020) during the frequent knee movements that include walking, jogging, running, squatting, ascending and descending stairs, and transitioning from sitting to standing in daily life.

The patellar tendon attaches to the inferior pole of the patella and inserts into the tibia at the tibial tubercle. A plica is a fold in the membrane of the knee joint and is a thick fibrotic tissue that can become irritated from overuse, causing pain, inflammation, and, at times, instability at the knee joint.

FUNCTIONS OF THE KNEE JOINT

The important functions of the knee joint include weight bearing, mobility, stability, and shock absorption for the forces that occur from the feet during walking and running.

The knee joint plays a significant role in maintaining balance and stability of the body. Stability at the knee joint can be classified into static and dynamic. Static stability is the ability to maintain a stable position while standing, while dynamic stability refers to the ability to maintain stability while moving. Static stability is provided by the ligaments, the menisci, and the articular surfaces. Dynamic stability is derived from the muscular attachments around the knee joint. The knee joint works in conjunction with the hip and ankle joints to allow us to walk, run, and jump. The knee joint also allows for a small amount of rotation, which is important for activities such as pivoting and turning.

Weight bearing is one of the chief functions of the knee joint. The knee joint supports the weight of the upper body and plays a crucial role in maintaining balance and stability. The knee joint is designed in such a way as to bear weight and withstand the forces caused by movement and impact. The anterior cruciate ligament (ACL), posterior cruciate ligament (PCL), medial collateral ligament (MCL), and lateral collateral ligament (LCL) work together to provide appropriate stability and prevent excessive movement at the joint. Additionally, the knee joint is reinforced by the patella, which helps to distribute forces across the joint.

The knee joint also plays a key role in shock absorption. When we walk or run, the knee joint absorbs the impact of each step, reducing the stress on other parts of the body such as the spine and hips. This is achieved by the knee joint's ability to flex and extend, which allows it to function as a shock absorber by absorbing and distributing the impact of each step we take.

In addition to its mechanical functions, the knee joint is also involved in several physiological processes (Smith, 2019). The knee joint is rich in sensory receptors, which provide important feedback to the brain about the position and movement of the joint (Jones, 2018). This feedback is crucial for maintaining balance and coordination, as well as for controlling movement and preventing injury (Brown, 2017). The knee joint is also innervated by several nerves, including the femoral nerve, which is responsible for providing sensation to the front of the thigh (Johnson, 2016), and the sciatic nerve, which is responsible for providing sensation to the back of the thigh and leg (Williams, 2015).

The knee joint also plays a vital role in proprioception. Proprioception is the ability of an individual to sense the position and movement of the body in relation to space. The knee joint helps in proprioception by means of receptors located in the ligaments, tendons, and muscles that surround the joint. These receptors send signals to the brain, thus enabling the body to sense the position and movement of the knee joint, thus allowing for precise control of movement. The popliteal artery is responsible for supplying blood to the lower leg, and it is crucial for maintaining the health and function of the knee joint (Bowers Z et al. 2022).

Injuries to the knee joint can occur from various causes such as overuse, trauma, and degenerative conditions. Overuse injuries, such as runner's knee, can occur from repetitive stress on the knee joint and are commonly noticed in athletes. Traumatic injuries, such as a ligament tear, commonly occur from sudden impacts or twists. Degenerative conditions such as osteoarthritis usually occur from wear and tear on the joint over a period of time.

ROLE OF THE KNEE JOINT IN THE GAIT CYCLE (WALKING CYCLE)

The knee joint plays a crucial role in the gait cycle, particularly during the stance phase. The sequence of movements occurring in the body when one moves through a complete stride or step during walking or running is called the gait cycle.

In humans, walking can be divided into the stance and swing phases. The stance phase is when the foot is in contact with the ground and classified as four sub-phases namely the heel strike, loading response, mid-stance and toe-off. The swing phase is when the foot is off the ground and classified in two sub-phases, namely the initial swing, midswing, and terminal swing. The stance phase accounts for 65% of the gait cycle, while the swing phase accounts for 35% (Zhang et al., 2020).

The major muscles acting on the knee joint comprise the quadriceps and the hamstrings. The quadriceps lie anterior to the femur and the knee, while the hamstrings lie posterior. The quadriceps work together to straighten the knee, while the hamstrings bend the knee. The gastrocnemius and soleus muscles in the calf also contribute to knee movement.

STANCE PHASE

Heel-strike

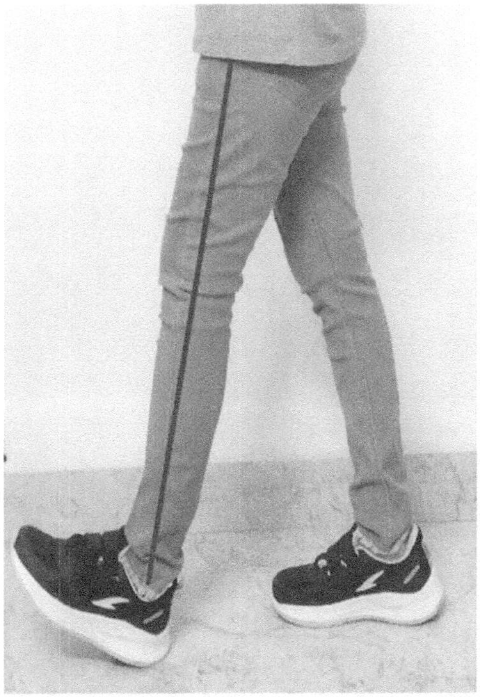

Loading response

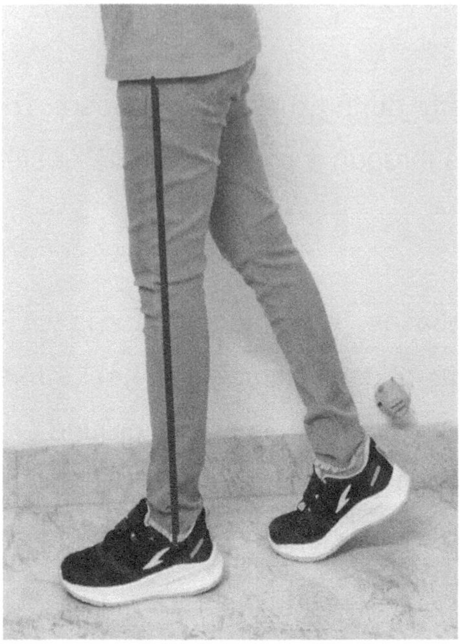

Midstance

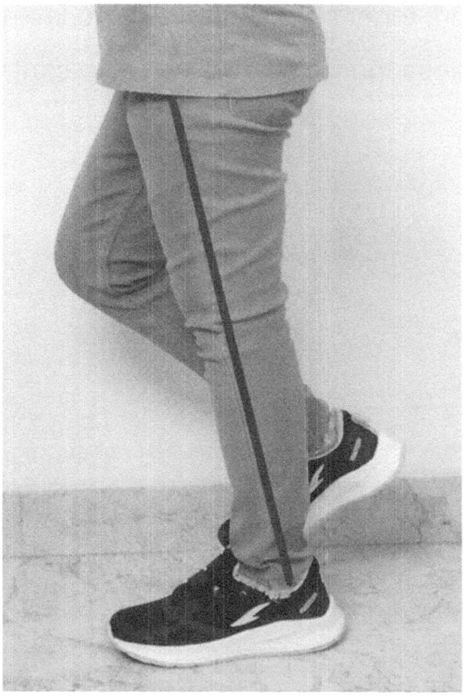

Toe off

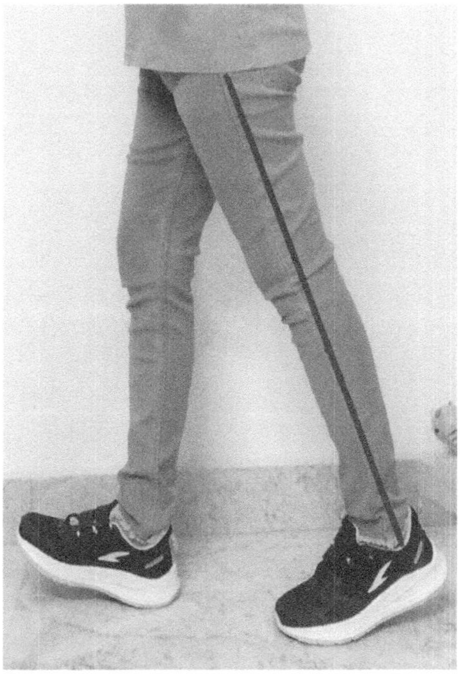

SWING PHASE

Initial Swing

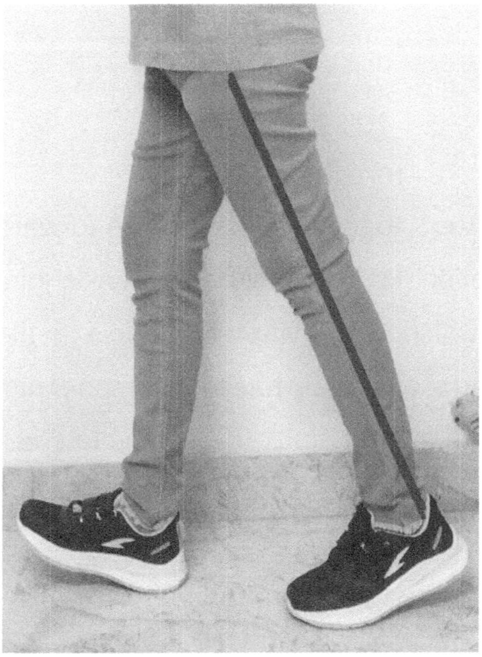

Mid Swing

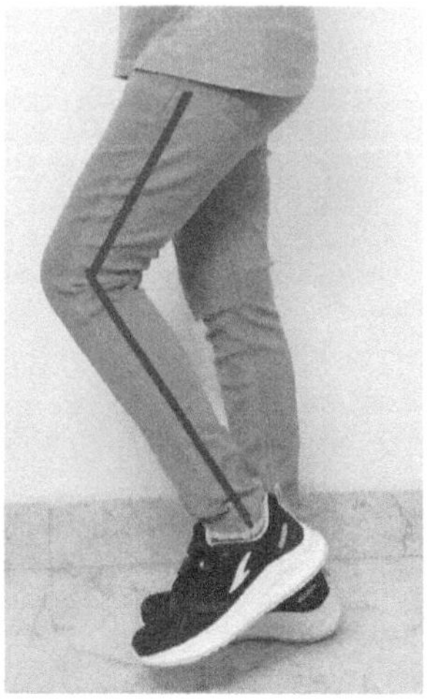

Terminal Swing

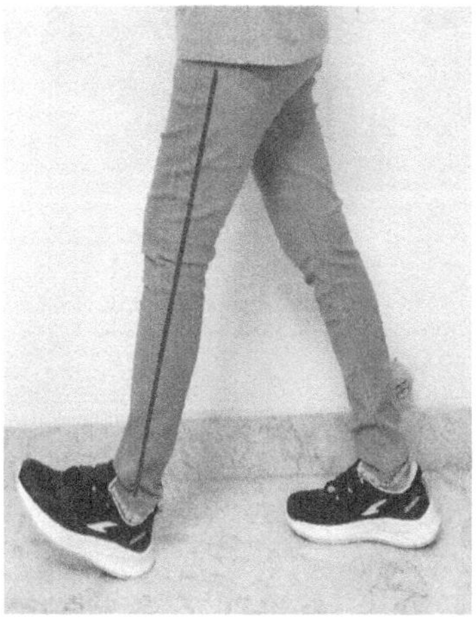

During walking, the muscles around the knee, ankle, and foot work together to control the forward movement of the body. The quadriceps, patellofemoral articulation, tibialis anterior, and ankle joint all play a role in slowing down the body during the part of the walking cycle when the foot is on the ground, called the stance phase (Chhabra et al., 2001). The quadriceps group has four components: the rectus femoris, vastus medialis, vastus lateralis, and vastus intermedius. The vastus lateralis constitutes about 50% of the muscle mass in the quadriceps group.

Muscles of the knee joint

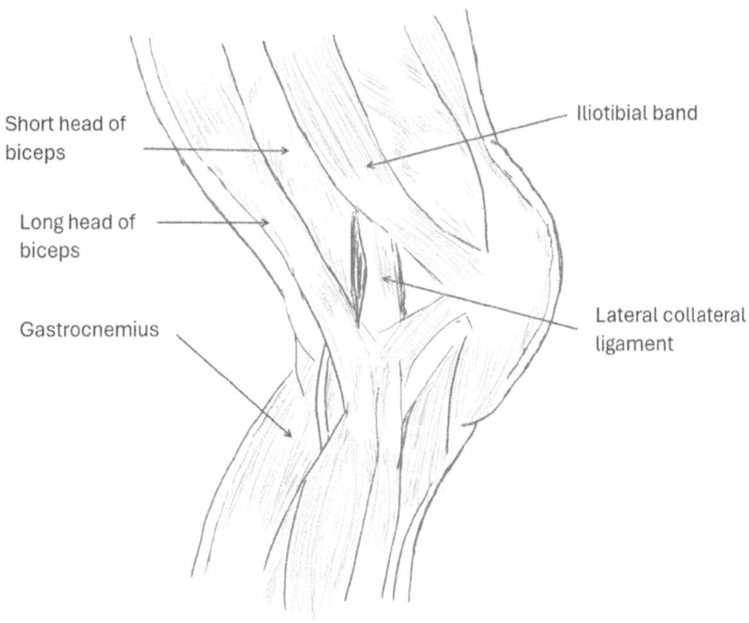

The knee joint allows for flexion and extension, which is necessary for the forward propulsion of the body during walking or running (Perry, 1992). During this phase, the knee joint is responsible for absorbing shock as the foot strikes the ground, as well as providing the propulsion needed for forward motion (Smith et al., 2018). Propulsion occurs by extending the leg and pushing off the ground (Perry, 1992). This is done with the aid of the quadriceps and hamstring muscles (Perry, 1992). The knee joint also plays a role in the swing phase (Perry, 1992), as it flexes to clear the ground during the forward motion of the leg (Perry, 1992).

During the stance phase, the knee joint undergoes flexion and extension, allowing the foot to contact the ground and then push off again. The knee joint also controls the rotation of the lower leg, thus helping to maintain balance and stability during the gait cycle.

Proper function of the knee joint is essential for normal gait, and any dysfunction or injury can result in gait abnormalities and pain (Brown et al., 2019). For example, knee osteoarthritis, a degenerative joint disease, can lead to difficulty in walking and reduce the ability of the knee joint to absorb shock and bear weight.

CAUSES AND RISK FACTORS OF KNEE ARTHRITIS

Knee arthritis is a condition that affects the knee joint, causing pain, stiffness and difficulty with mobility. This book focuses in detail on the arthritis of the knee due to cartilage degeneration and cartilage injuries.

There are several risk factors that can increase the likelihood of developing knee arthritis. These include:

1. **Ageing:** Ageing is the most common factor subjecting the cartilage to wear and tear, leading to arthritis. This is commonly known as osteoarthritis, the most common form of arthritis in the knee. The prevalence of osteoarthritis increases with age, and it is estimated that about 9.6% of men and 18% of women aged 60 years or over have symptomatic knee osteoarthritis (WHO, 2020).

2. **Injury:** Any previous injuries to the knee, such as a fracture, sprains, or strains, can increase the risk of developing arthritis later in life. A study conducted by Roos et al. (2010) showed that individuals who had suffered a previous knee injury had a four-fold increased risk of developing knee osteoarthritis. Thus, people who have had cartilage injuries in the knee joint are at an increased risk of developing osteoarthritis in the affected joint.

3. **Overuse:** Repetitive stress on the knee, as in activities such as running or cycling, can lead to arthritis in later life. Individuals in certain professions, such as sports, are more prone to overuse injuries. According to a study by Felson et al. (1988), the risk of developing knee osteoarthritis increases with the increase in the number of miles run per week.

4. **Obesity:** People who are overweight or obese often develop arthritis due to the extra stress on their knee joints. A study conducted by Felson et al. (1988) found that individuals with a body mass index (BMI) of thirty or higher had a fourfold increased risk of developing knee osteoarthritis.

5. **Genetics:** It is believed that certain genetic variations may cause a person to be more susceptible to arthritis. Certain genetic mutations and variations, such as the COL2A1,

COL11A1, and COMP genes, may predispose a person to an increased risk of knee arthritis. A study by Jordan et al. (2000) found that individuals with a family history of knee osteoarthritis had a two-fold increased risk of developing the condition.

Preventing knee pain begins with maintaining a healthy weight, as extra weight can put extra stress on the knee joint (Mayo Clinic, 2020). Stretching and strengthening exercises, particularly for the quadriceps and hamstrings, can also help to support and protect the knee joint (American Academy of Orthopaedic Surgeons, 2019). Wearing appropriate shoes and using proper form and technique during physical activities can also help to reduce the risk of knee injury and pain (Mayo Clinic, 2020).

COMMON CONDITIONS AFFECTING THE KNEE JOINT

The knee is a complex joint that is vulnerable to a variety of pathological conditions that can lead to pain (American Academy of Orthopaedic Surgeons, 2019). Some of the most common causes of knee pain include osteoarthritis, rheumatoid arthritis, meniscal tears, ligament tears (such as ACL or MCL tears), tendonitis, bursitis, and patellofemoral pain syndrome.

Osteoarthritis is a degenerative condition that occurs when the cartilage in the knee joint wears down over time (NIAMS health information on osteoarthritis 2022).

Meniscal tears are tears in the cartilage that acts as a cushion between the thigh bone and shinbone (American Academy of Orthopaedic Surgeons, 2019). These tears can occur due to injury or degeneration and can cause pain, swelling, and difficulty moving the joint.

Ligament tears, such as ACL or MCL tears, occur when the ligaments that support the knee joint are stretched or torn (American Academy of Orthopaedic Surgeons, 2019). These tears can occur due to injury, such as from a sudden twist or impact, and can cause severe pain, swelling, and difficulty bearing weight on the affected leg.

Tendonitis is inflammation of the tendons that attach the muscles to the bones in the knee (Mayo Clinic, 2020). This can cause pain, tenderness, and difficulty moving the joint.

Bursitis is inflammation of the fluid-filled sacs (bursa) that cushion the knee joint, which can lead to pain, swelling, and stiffness (Mayo Clinic, 2020).

Patellofemoral pain syndrome is a condition that occurs when the kneecap (patella) rubs against the thigh bone (femur) instead of sliding smoothly over it (American Academy of Orthopaedic Surgeons, 2019). This can lead to pain, discomfort, and difficulty moving the knee.

Rheumatoid arthritis (RA): Knee arthritis is a common symptom in individuals suffering from rheumatoid arthritis. This is an autoimmune disorder that is characterised by the body's own immune system attacking the lining of the joints, causing inflammation and pain. This type of arthritis can affect multiple joints in the body, including the knee and hip. Early diagnosis plays an important role in managing this condition effectively.

Gout: Gout is another type of arthritis characterised by the build-up of uric acid crystals in the joint, causing inflammation and pain. Usually, the first symptoms occur in the great toe. Other joints can eventually be involved. A study by Zhu and colleagues in 2015 suggested gout may increase the likelihood of developing knee osteoarthritis in later life.

Psoriatic arthritis: This is a form of arthritis that occurs in people with psoriasis, a skin condition characterised by red, scaly patches. It's been reported by the National Psoriasis Foundation that a significant portion of individuals living with psoriasis, as much as 30%, may also experience psoriatic arthritis, a form of arthritis that develops in some people with psoriasis.

Baker's cyst: A fluid-filled cyst that can form behind the knee and cause pain and swelling (Mayo Clinic, 2020).

In addition to these specific conditions, knee pain can also be caused by overuse or injury, such as from playing sports or engaging in repetitive motions (American Academy of Orthopaedic Surgeons, 2019). Other risk factors for knee pain include obesity, poor posture, and muscle imbalances (Mayo Clinic, 2020).

SYMPTOMS OF KNEE ARTHRITIS

Knee arthritis due to cartilage issues occurs frequently and may disrupt one's daily life due to discomfort, pain, inflammation, and restriction of movements in the affected joint. Cartilage, a connective tissue, is found in various parts of the body. It is elastic in nature and commonly found at bone ends, allowing the smooth movement of the bones.

Multiple injuries indicate that cartilage injuries may cause arthritis in the long term. Hence, it becomes important to treat cartilage injuries at the earliest. This was emphasised by the study that was published in the journal 'Osteoarthritis and Cartilage,' in which 657 patients who underwent surgery for cartilage repair were followed for an average of 10 years. The study results showed about 48% of patients developed OA knee (Crema M.D., et al. 2010). A similar study by Guermazi, A. et al. (2011), published in the journal 'Arthritis Care and Research,' also indicated a higher risk of knee arthritis over time in patients with cartilage injuries, indicating the need for joint replacements.

There are several types of cartilage injuries that can occur in the knee joint, including fractures, meniscal tears, articular cartilage injuries, and osteochondritis dissecans. In severe cases, the joint may become swollen and deformed.

Symptoms of cartilage injuries in the knee joint commonly include:

- Pain that may increase with activity
- Swelling
- Stiffness
- Restriction in the range of movement
- A popping or snapping sound when the knee is bent or extended
- A feeling of instability in the knee or giving way

Rehabilitation for cartilage injuries will depend on the nature and severity of the injury. For minor injuries, such as a small meniscal tear, rest, ice, and physical therapy may be enough to help the knee heal. For more severe injuries, such as a large meniscal tear or a fracture, surgery may be necessary to repair the injury. Surgical procedures are explained in more detail in the later part of the book.

Pain is the most common symptom of knee arthritis. The pain can be felt in the knee joint and may be described by the patient as a dull ache or a sharp, stabbing sensation. The pain may be worse in the morning or after sitting for prolonged periods and may improve with movements. Pain may become constant as the condition of the affected knee worsens (American Academy of Orthopaedic Surgeons, 2021).

Stiffness is another complaint in patients affected by knee arthritis. The stiffness often tends to be worse in the morning, making it difficult to bend or straighten the knee. But when the individual may find the symptoms go away with movement, such as walking. The stiffness may last for a few minutes or a few hours and may improve with activity. (Arthritis Foundation, 2021)

Swelling and inflammation in the knee may make the affected knee feel warm to the touch and may appear red and swollen. As the condition worsens, the knee may become swollen even when one is not active. (Mayo Clinic, 2021). The warmth in the affected joint is due to the increased blood supply to the area. The more the blood supply, the more the oxygen and nutrition to the area, which is a part of the healing process.

Reduced range of motion in the knee interferes with activities in daily life. The knee may be stiff and difficult to bend or straighten, making it difficult to perform everyday activities such as climbing stairs or getting in and out of a car.

A popping or crunching sound or sensation in the knee joint can be caused by the degeneration of the cartilage in the joint and may indicate arthritis in more advanced stages.

Weakness or instability (feeling of giving way in the knee) in the knee can also be a symptom of knee arthritis for some patients. The knee may feel wobbly or unsteady, making it difficult to walk or stand. This can be caused by the degeneration of the cartilage in the joint and may indicate an advanced condition of arthritis.

In addition to these symptoms, individuals with knee arthritis may also have trouble sleeping due to pain and stiffness in the knee. They may also have a decreased ability to participate in physical activities and exercise, which can lead to a decrease in overall physical fitness and an increase in the risk of other health problems.

Symptoms of knee arthritis

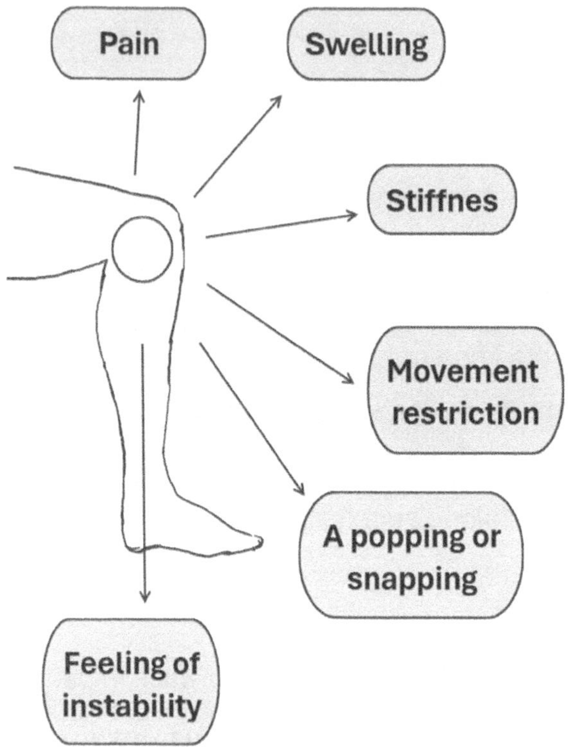

PHYSIOLOGY OF PAIN PERCEPTION

The Pain gate theory proposes that the perception of pain is modulated by the activity of certain nerve fibres, namely the A-delta and C fibres in the spinal cord. According to the theory, these nerve fibres act as a "gate" that can be opened or closed by various physiological and psychological factors. According to the theory, the gate is controlled by two types of nerve fibres: A-beta, the large, myelinated fibres that carry non-painful sensations such as touch and pressure, and A-delta and C-fibres, the small, unmyelinated fibres that carry painful sensations.

The theory suggests that when the "gate" is open, pain signals are allowed to travel to the brain, and when it is closed, the signals are blocked, and the person may not experience pain. The pain gate theory, also known as the "gate control theory of pain," was first proposed by Ronald Melzack and Patrick Wall in 1965. For example, when rubbing a sore spot on your body, the pressure and touch sensations from the rubbing activates the large fibres and closes the gate to the small fibres that carry pain signals, thus reducing the pain perception.

The pain gate theory has been supported by many studies and has been found to be a useful tool for understanding and managing pain in patients, especially with chronic pain. Based on the pain gate theory, several pain management techniques have been come into use, such as spinal cord stimulation and transcutaneous electrical nerve stimulation (TENS), which make use of electrical impulses to activate large fibres and to close the gate to small fibres.

The brain can also modulate pain perception through the release of certain neurotransmitters and hormones, such as endorphins and serotonin.

Other theories of pain include the pain neuromatrix theory and the biopsychosocial model of pain. The Neuromatrix model of pain suggests that pain is a complex and multidimensional experience that is created by the interaction of various neural, psychological, and social factors. The biopsychosocial model of pain emphasises the role of psychological and social factors in pain perception and pain management.

The Pain Gate Theory

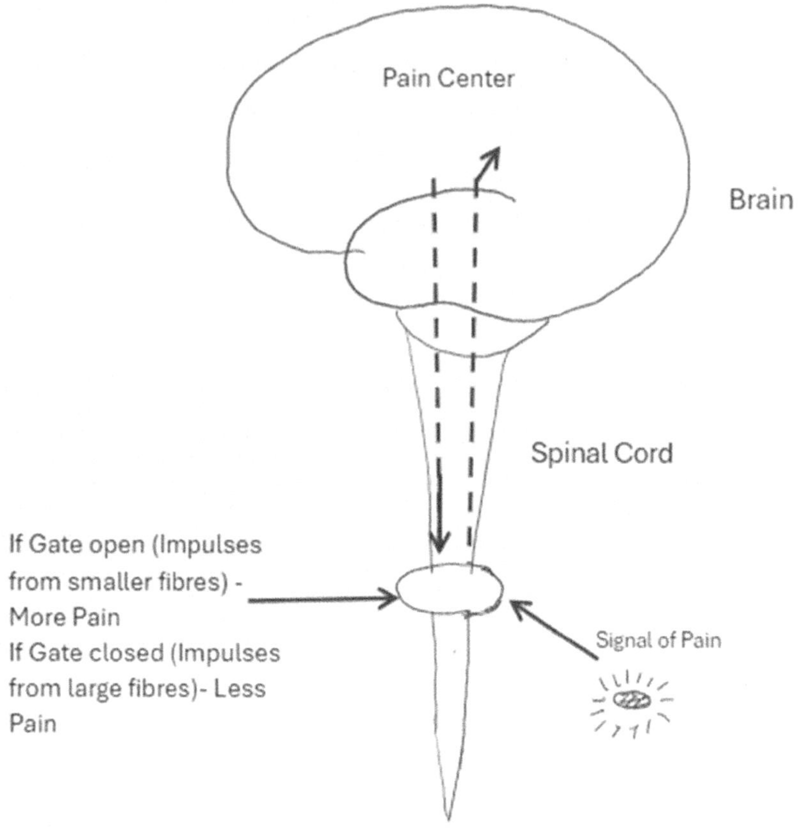

The pain management strategies, such as cognitive-behavioural therapy (CBT) and mindfulness-based interventions, can help in reducing the pain perception in individuals and in better management of daily life. CBT is a form of psychotherapy that works by helping patients change their thoughts, behaviours, and emotions related to pain and has been found to be effective in reducing chronic pain. Mindfulness-based interventions, such as mindfulness-based stress reduction (MBSR) and mindfulness-based cognitive therapy (MBCT), also help to reduce pain by teaching individuals how to focus their attention on the present moment and thus disengage from their negative thoughts and emotions that may exacerbate pain.

PHYSICAL THERAPY ASSESSMENT OF THE KNEE JOINT

Diagnosis of knee pain typically begins with a physical examination, during which the Doctor will examine the knee and check for signs of swelling, tenderness, and instability (American Academy of Orthopaedic Surgeons, 2019). They may also test range of motion and reflexes. Imaging tests, such as X-rays, MRI, or CT scans, may also be ordered to help determine the cause of the pain and rule out any serious conditions (Mayo Clinic, 2020).

ASSESSMENT OF THE KNEE JOINT

The physiotherapist will perform a thorough assessment of the affected knee joint, including range of motion, strength, stability, and any associated pain or discomfort and will regularly re-evaluate the patient's progress and adjust the treatment plan as needed.

The assessment protocol for the knee joint in knee arthritis by a physical therapist typically involves the following steps:

Subjective Assessment: The therapist will ask the patient about their medical history, symptoms, and overall functional abilities. This will help the therapist understand the patient's needs and goals for physiotherapy. This can include:

> **Medical History:** The therapist will ask about the patient's history of knee pain or injury, as well as any other medical conditions that may affect the knee joint.
> **Symptoms:** The therapist will ask the patient to describe their current symptoms, including the location of pain, intensity, and duration of any pain or discomfort in the knee joint.
> **Functional Limitations:** The therapist will ask the patient about their overall functional abilities, including any difficulties with daily activities, such as walking, climbing stairs, or getting in and out of a chair.

History of previous treatment: Any previous treatment undertaken by the patient including the knee pain, medications used, surgery undertaken, and Physical therapy.

Goals: The therapist will ask the patient to identify their goals for physiotherapy, such as reducing pain, improving mobility, or returning to specific activities. This information will guide the development of an individualised treatment plan and also help in understanding patients better.

The objective assessment for the knee joint involves observing and testing the patient's physical abilities and knee joint condition. This can include:

Observations: The therapist will then observe the patient's gait (walking pattern), posture, and movements to check the extent of any limitations or asymmetries (in case of abnormal postures).

Palpation: The therapist will feel for any tenderness, swelling, or deformities in the knee joint using their hands for evaluation.

The following are the common palpation techniques used to evaluate the knee joint:

Soft Tissue Palpation: The therapist will feel for any tenderness or swelling in the soft tissues surrounding the knee joint, including the quadriceps, hamstrings, and calf muscles.

Joint Line Palpation: The therapist will locate the joint line of the knee (the point at which the bones of the knee come together) and check for any tenderness or swelling in this area.

Bony Landmark Palpation: The therapist will feel for any deformities or abnormalities in the bones of the knee, including the femur, tibia, and patella.

Meniscal Palpation: The therapist may perform a few special tests, such as the McMurray test, to assess for any damage to the knee's meniscus, cartilage that helps absorb shock in the knee joint.

Range of Motion Assessment: The therapist will assess the patient's ability to move the knee joint through its full range of motion, including flexion and extension, and evaluate for any pain or stiffness.

Patellar Tracking Assessment: The therapist may assess the movement of the patella (kneecap) as the knee moves through its range of motion to identify any abnormal tracking patterns.

These techniques will help the therapist identify any areas of tenderness, swelling, or deformity in the knee joint and determine if these are contributing to the patient's symptoms. The results of the palpation will be used in combination with the patient's subjective information and other objective assessments to develop a comprehensive understanding of the patient's knee joint condition.

Strength Assessment: The therapist will assess the strength of the muscles surrounding the knee joint, including the quadriceps and hamstrings, as well as the muscles around the hip joint to determine if any weakness is contributing to the patient's symptoms.

The following are common strength assessments used to evaluate the knee joint:

Quadriceps Strength Assessment: The therapist will assess the strength of the quadriceps muscle group, which is responsible for knee extension, by having the patient perform exercises such as straight leg raises.

Hamstring Strength Assessment: The therapist will assess the strength of the hamstrings, which are responsible for knee flexion, by having the patient perform exercises such as hamstring curls.

Calf Strength Assessment: The therapist will assess the strength of the calf muscles, including the gastrocnemius and soleus, by having the patient perform exercises such as calf raises.

Isometric Testing: The therapist may have the patient perform isometric exercises, in which there is muscle contraction but without movement, to assess strength and stability in specific positions. Abnormalities in strength can indicate a need for specific exercises or interventions to improve muscle function and reduce the risk of future injury.

Stability Assessment: The therapist will assess the stability of the knee joint, including the ability to maintain balance and perform functional movements.

Stability assessment is an important part of evaluating the knee joint, as instability can be a major factor in knee pain and injury. The following are common stability assessments used by physical therapists:

Static Stability Assessment: The therapist will assess the patient's ability to maintain balance while standing still or performing simple movements, such as standing on one leg or shifting weight from one foot to the other.

Dynamic stability assessment: The therapist will assess the patient's ability to maintain stability while performing more complex movements, such as jumping, or hopping.

Ligament stability assessment: The therapist may perform specific tests, such as the Lachman test or the anterior drawer test, to assess the stability of the knee's ligaments, which are responsible for maintaining knee stability.

Special Tests: Special tests are a set of examination procedures used by physical therapists to evaluate specific aspects of knee joint function and identify the underlying cause of knee pain or injury. The therapist may perform special tests, such as the McMurray test or the Apley compression test, to assess the knee joint for specific conditions or to help diagnose knee arthritis.

The following are some common special tests used for the knee joint:

McMurray Test: This test is used to assess for meniscal injuries in the knee joint. The therapist will apply pressure to the knee while the patient's knee is passively rotated and flexed (bent), looking for any pain or clicking sensations.

Apley's Compression Test: This test is used in the assessment of knee joint pain and instability. The therapist will apply pressure to the knee while the patient's knee is passively flexed and extended, looking for any pain or instability.

Thessaly Test: This test is used to identify patellofemoral pain syndrome, a common condition affecting the knee joint. The therapist will have the patient perform a squatting movement while observing the patella (kneecap) for any abnormal tracking or pain.

Lachman Test: This test is used to assess the stability of the anterior cruciate ligament (ACL) in the knee joint. The therapist will apply a sudden anterior force to the knee while the patient's knee is flexed to 20-30 degrees, looking for any excessive movement or instability.

Anterior Drawer Test: This test is used to assess the stability of the anterior cruciate ligament (ACL) in the knee joint. The therapist will apply a sudden anterior force to the knee while the patient's knee is flexed to 90 degrees, looking for any excessive movement or instability.

Imaging: Imaging studies, such as X-rays or MRI, are used to further evaluate the extent of knee joint damage and to guide treatment planning.

The results of the objective assessment will be used in combination with the patient's subjective information to develop a comprehensive understanding of the patient's knee joint condition and guide the development of an individualised treatment plan.

PHYSICAL THERAPY MANAGEMENT IN KNEE ARTHRITIS

Exercise is a key component of physical therapy for cartilage injuries. Gentle range-of-motion exercises, such as knee flexion and extension, can help to maintain joint mobility and prevent stiffness. Strengthening exercises, such as leg presses and leg extensions, can help to improve muscle function and support the joint.

In addition, balance and proprioception exercises, such as single-leg stance and balance board exercises, can help to improve stability and coordination and prevent falls.

Manual therapy such as joint mobilisation and soft tissue mobilisation can also be helpful in improving range of motion, reducing pain, and promoting healing.

Physical therapy management also includes education on proper body mechanics and activity modification to prevent re-injury and enhance healing.

Treatment for knee pain will vary depending on the underlying cause but may include rest, physical therapy, exercises to strengthen the muscles that support the knee, and medications to reduce pain and inflammation (American Academy of Orthopaedic Surgeons, 2019). In some cases, a brace or splint may be recommended to provide support to the joint. Surgery may be recommended for severe or persistent knee pain, especially for conditions such as ACL or meniscal tears that may require repair or reconstruction (American Academy of Orthopaedic Surgeons, 2019).

Regular exercise is an important aspect of managing knee arthritis and benefits the individual by reducing pain, improving joint mobility, and increasing muscle strength and endurance. Now let us briefly go through some of the studies that indicate the role of exercises in improving knee pain, function, and mobility.

A study published in the Journal of Rheumatology showed that a 12-week program of quadriceps strengthening exercises led to significant improvements in knee pain and function in patients with knee osteoarthritis. The study participants included patients with moderate-to-severe knee osteoarthritis and performed exercises such as leg presses and knee extensions three times per week. They reported a decrease in pain and an improvement in physical function. The results were measured using the Western Ontario and McMaster Universities Osteoarthritis Index (WOMAC) scale.

A similar study, published in the Journal of Orthopaedic and Sports Physical Therapy, found that a 12-week program of aerobic and resistance exercises in patients with mild to moderate osteoarthritis was effective in reducing pain and improving function in the knee joint. The study participants performed exercises such as cycling, stair climbing, and leg press three times per week. They also reported a significant improvement in their physical function according to the results measured by the WOMAC scale.

Another similar study published by the Journal of Physical Therapy Science also indicated that range of motion exercises are very effective in improving joint mobility and reducing pain in patients with knee osteoarthritis through a 12-week program.

ACUTE REHABILITATION

Physical therapy plays a critical role in the acute rehabilitation of cartilage injuries. The initial protocol of physical therapy during the acute phase is to control pain and inflammation, protect the injured tissue, and promote healing.

To reduce pain and inflammation, Physical therapists may use modalities such as ice, ultrasound, and electrical stimulation. They also help in reducing muscle spasms and improving the range of motion. Splints and braces may also help protect the affected joint by restricting movement and preventing any further injury at the affected joint.

Aquatic therapy (hydrotherapy) can be an effective option for patients with cartilage injuries, as the buoyancy of the water can help to reduce stress on the joint and provide an ideal environment for exercise.

Patients are educated on the nature of their injury, the importance of rest and proper medication, the performance of appropriate exercises, and the proper use of assistive devices such as crutches and canes.

REHABILITATION IN THE SUBACUTE AND CHRONIC PHASE

In the subacute phase (1-4 weeks post-injury), the main goals of physical therapy are to reduce pain and inflammation, protect the injured area, and begin to restore range of motion. This may include the use of modalities such as ice, ultrasound, and electrical stimulation, as well as exercises to improve joint mobility and muscle strength.

As the injury progresses to the chronic phase (greater than 4 weeks post-injury), the focus of physical therapy shifts to improving joint function and muscle strength and preventing the development of secondary complications such as muscle imbalances and joint stiffness. This may include exercises to improve range of motion, increase strength, and improve coordination, as well as the use of therapeutic modalities such as heat, exercises, and manual therapy.

The complete recovery of cartilage injuries may take a few weeks to several months, but with appropriate management of these injuries, the patients may regain their normal activities with minimal long-term complications. Physical therapists may also incorporate balance exercises and proprioception training, as cartilage injury can affect the stability and control of the joint.

MANAGING PAIN AND INFLAMMATION

MEDICATIONS

Most commonly medications used to manage the symptoms of knee arthritis are as follows:

Acetaminophen: This medication relieves pain and reduces fever. It is considered safe for most people to use and is often recommended when the non-pharmacological interventions are not effective. Acetaminophen can cause liver damage if taken in large doses; hence, it should be used according to the package instructions and strictly under Physician's advice.

Nonsteroidal Anti-Inflammatory Drugs (NSAIDs): These medications, such as Ibuprofen and Naproxen, are also used to relieve pain and reduce inflammation in the body. They should be used under Physician's guidance. Care should be taken to use them according to the package instructions and not exceed the recommended dosage. Long-term use of NSAIDs may cause stomach ulcers and kidney problems and may cause other side effects. People with heart disease, high blood pressure, or bleeding disorders should be especially careful when using these medications and consult Physicians before use (Arthritis Foundation).

Glucosamine and chondroitin: These are supplements that are often used to help alleviate knee arthritis pain and improve joint function. Glucosamine is a natural compound and helps to build and repair cartilage. Chondroitin is a naturally found carbohydrate that helps in decreasing inflammation. These supplements should be used carefully and after proper healthcare consultation, and also these supplements may cause severe allergic reactions in some, especially for those who are allergic to shellfish and other seafood.

Omega-3 fatty acids: Omega-3 fatty acids are a type of healthy fat that can help reduce inflammation and improve joint function. Fish oil supplements are a good source of omega-3s.

Even though some OTC medications can help manage the symptoms of knee arthritis, they may not help the underlying cause of the condition. It is also important to consult with a doctor before starting any new medication, especially if the patient has other comorbidities or is taking any other medications.

TOPICAL CREAMS AND GELS

There are several OTC topical creams and gels that can be used for knee arthritis to relieve pain and reduce inflammation. These include products that most often contain menthol, capsaicin, and salicylates. These products can provide localised pain relief but may not be as effective as oral medications (Healthline, n.d.).

Topical creams and gels are products that are applied directly to the skin to provide localised pain relief and to reduce inflammation. Some of the most used topical creams and gels for knee arthritis include:

1. **Menthol:** This is a naturally occurring compound that is derived from mint plants. It has a cooling sensation occurring applied to the skin, which can provide pain relief. Menthol works by activating a specific type of cold receptor in the skin, which blocks the transmission of pain signals to the brain (NCCIH, n.d.).

2. **Capsaicin:** This is a compound that is found in chilli peppers. A substance, substance P, is responsible for the transmission of pain signals to the brain (NCCIH). Capsaicin works by depleting this substance.

3. **Salicylates:** These compounds that are related to aspirin and are found in several plants, such as willow bark. They work by reducing inflammation and pain (NCCIH, n.d.).

4. **Camphor:** This compound is derived from the wood of the camphor tree. It has a cooling and soothing effect when applied to the skin and can provide pain relief (WebMD, n.d.).

5. **Counterirritants:** These compounds cause a mild irritation when applied to the skin and can provide pain relief by distracting the brain from the pain in the knee joint (WebMD, n.d.). Examples of counterirritants include methyl salicylate, which is found in many muscle creams, and menthol.

Topical creams and gels can provide localised pain relief and reduce inflammation but do not address the underlying cause of knee arthritis. People with sensitive skin or allergies should be especially careful when using these products and should test a small amount of the cream or gel on a small patch of skin before using it on the knee.

HEAT AND COLD THERAPY

HEAT THERAPY

Heat therapy is a form of treatment that uses heat to increase blood flow, relax muscles, and reduce pain and stiffness in the knee joint caused by arthritis (Arthritis Foundation, n.d.). There are several types of heat therapy that can be used to manage knee arthritis, including:

1. **Moist heat therapy:** This type of heat therapy uses water or a damp cloth to create heat. Moist heat is more effective than dry heat because it penetrates deeper into the skin and muscles, which can provide more relief for knee arthritis pain (National Health Service, 2018). Moist heat can be applied using a heating pad, hot water bottle, or a damp towel that has been heated in the microwave.

2. **Dry heat therapy:** This type of heat therapy uses dry heat sources, such as a heating pad, electric blanket, or infrared lamp. Dry heat is less effective than moist heat because it does not penetrate as deeply into the skin and muscles (National Health Service, 2018). Dry heat can be applied for a longer period than moist heat without causing skin irritation.

3. **Paraffin wax bath:** This type of heat therapy uses warm paraffin wax to provide deep heat to the knee joint. The wax is heated and maintained at a temperature between 40-44 degree Celsius, and a lint localised piece can be dipped in paraffin wax and applied on the knee for 15-20 minutes at a time (National Health Service, 2018). Paraffin wax baths are particularly useful for people with arthritis in the hands and feet, as they can be used to cover the entire joint.

Electric Heating Pad

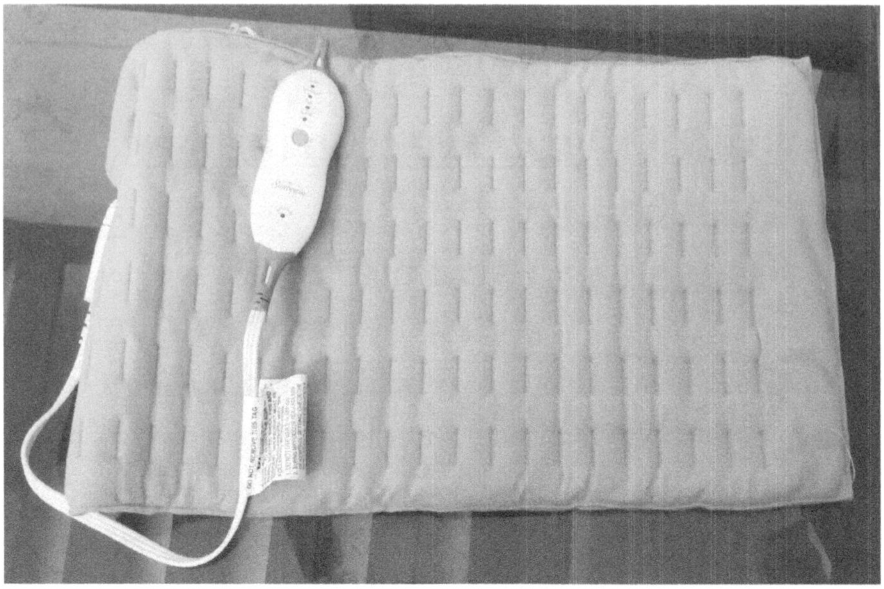

The Infrared Lamp

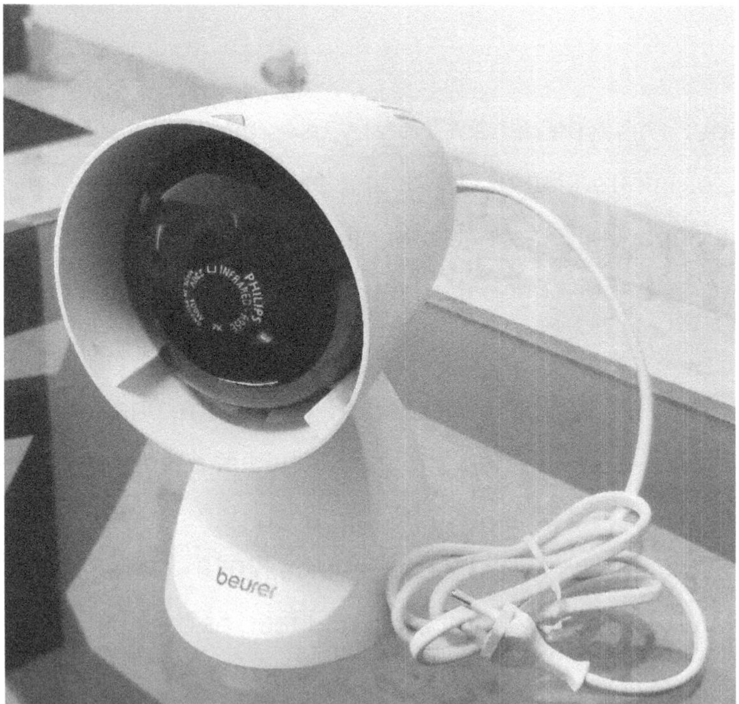

Heat therapy is contraindicated for people with poor circulation, diabetes, deep vein thrombosis, or a history of burns (Arthritis Foundation, n.d.). Heat therapy should be applied at a comfortable temperature and avoid overheating (National Health Service, 2018).

COLD THERAPY

Cold therapy, also known as cryotherapy, works by reducing blood flow to the affected area, which in turn reduces inflammation and numbs the area to provide pain relief. There are several types of cold therapy that can be used to manage knee arthritis, including:

1. **Ice packs:** Ice packs can be applied to the knee to provide localised cold therapy. The ice pack should be wrapped in a towel to protect the skin and should be applied for not more than 20 minutes at a time (with frequent breaks to avoid discomfort and injury to skin), with at least 40 minutes in between applications (Mayo Clinic, 2018).

2. **Cryotherapy:** Cryotherapy involves using a cold spray or cold gel to provide a more intense cooling effect than an ice pack. Cryotherapy should be applied for a shorter period (5-10 minutes) and should be used under the guidance of a healthcare professional (Mayo Clinic, 2018).

3. **Cold compresses:** Cold compresses can be made by soaking a cloth in cold water and wringing it out. The compress should be applied to the knee for 15-20 minutes at a time (Johns Hopkins Medicine, n.d.).

It's important to note that cold therapy should not be applied to the skin for more than 20 minutes at a time, as it can cause frostbite (Mayo Clinic, 2018). Cold therapy is contraindicated in patients with poor circulation at the affected area and should be used with utmost care and under medical supervision in patients with comorbidities.

THERAPEUTIC EXERCISES TO STRENGTHEN KNEE JOINT

EXERCISES IN LYING

The key to improving the function of the knee joint in patients suffering from arthritis is to find low-impact exercises that will not put too much stress on the knees. This can be achieved by incorporating exercises in a lying position so that there is little or no impact on the knee joints. This could help reduce stress on the knee joint.

The knee joint strength can be improved by incorporating various kinds of exercises targeting the different muscle groups in the lower limb, thus improving the overall quality of life of an individual.

Special note 1:

The individual should slowly progress with the exercises in lying, then ROM exercises, strengthening exercises, followed by resistance band exercises and then if comfortable with the knees (without aggravating the existing knee pain) should go ahead with the wall siled and squats.

Special note 2:

The information provided in this book is exclusively for individuals suffering with cartilage issues caused by injury and degenerative changes and not for the autoimmune related and similar conditions causing knee arthritis and pain. Individuals with autoimmune related disorders need more customized assessment and individualised treatment care which is not discussed in this book and will be added in the future editions.

STRETCHING OF MUSCLES AROUND KNEE JOINT

Before starting with exercises, it is crucial to perform warm-up and stretching for the muscles to avoid any injuries or soreness.

.

HAMSTRING STRETCH IN SITTING:

Sit on the floor with one leg (to be stretched) straight out in front of you and the other leg bent at the knee as shown in the picture below. Bend forward at the hips and reach towards your toes. Hold the stretch for 15-20 seconds and repeat 2-3 times on each leg.

Hamstring stretch

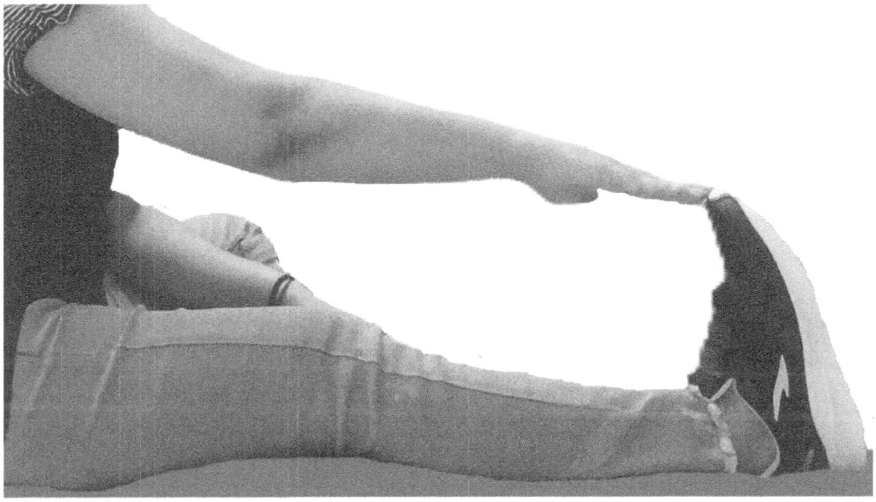

HAMSTRING STRETCH IN LYING:

The lying hamstring stretch can help stretch the muscles that run along the back of the thigh, the hamstrings, thus reducing tension on the knee joint. To perform this exercise, lie on your back with your legs straight and together. Slowly lift one leg up with the knee bent and then slowly straighten the knee towards the ceiling. Hold this position for 10-15 seconds, and then lower your leg back to the ground. Repeat this exercise 10-15 times for each leg.

Lying Hamstring Stretch

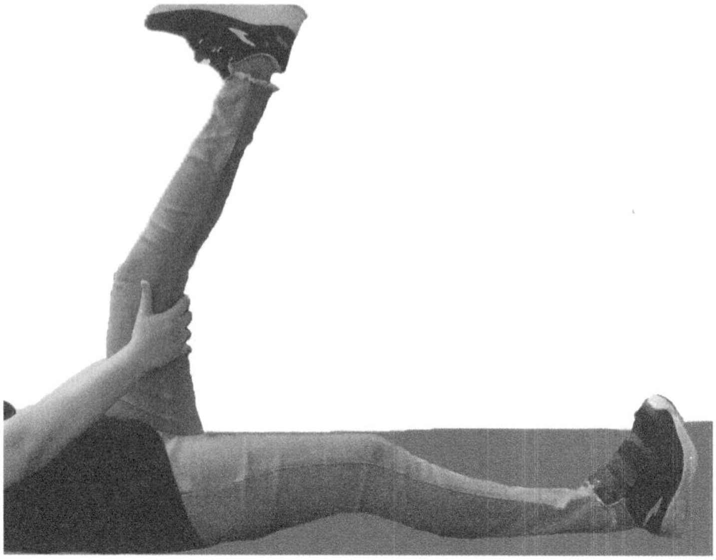

QUADRICEPS STRETCH IN LYING:

The quadriceps stretch (in lying) helps to stretch the muscles that run along the front side of the thigh, the quadriceps, thus reducing tension on the knee joint. To perform this exercise: By lying on the tummy with one hand under the forehead and the other hand under the hip, one can bend the knee and reach behind to hold the ankle with the hand (the one under the hip). The individual should hold this position for around 10-15 seconds and then let go. This stretch can be repeated 5 times for each leg.

Quadriceps stretch in lying

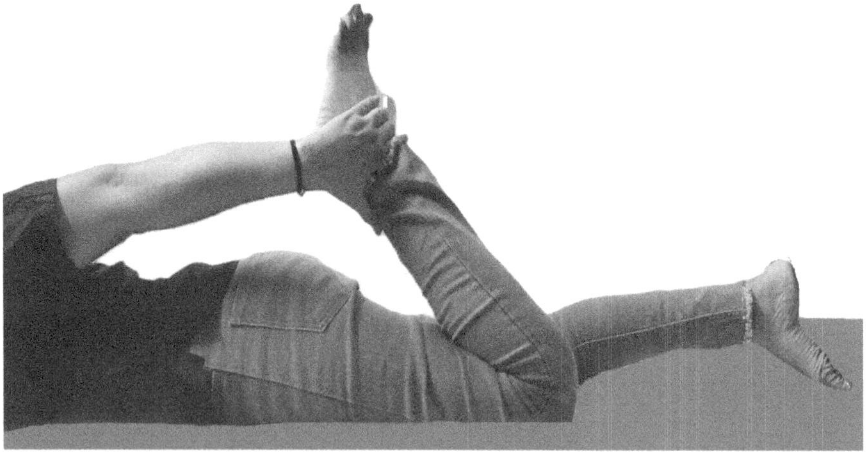

QUADRICEPS STRETCH IN STANDING:

If the individual is comfortable standing on one leg without hurting his knee, then the quadriceps stretch can also be performed in standing as shown in the picture below. Stand with your feet together and bend one knee, bringing your heel towards your buttocks. Take support from a wall to avoid a fall. Holding the ankle with one hand and pressing the hip forward for about 15-20 seconds. Repeat 2-3 times on each leg.

Quadriceps stretch in standing

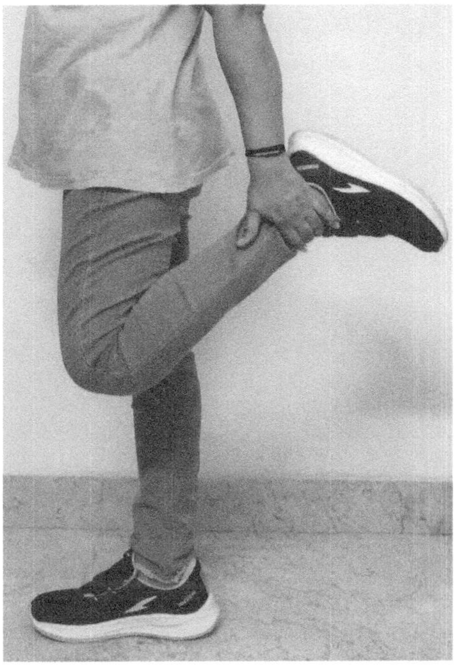

STATIC QUADRICEPS EXERCISE (QUAD SETS):

Static quadriceps exercises can be performed while lying on a bed. The individual can sit on the edge of the chair or else on the bed or floor with the legs extended in the front. By placing a towel or bedsheet rolled under the knee, the individual should flex his foot so that it points to the ceiling. Then the individual should gently press the knee down towards the floor on the towel roll, keeping the heel on the floor. This stretch is held for 15-20 seconds and 5 times for each session, then repeated for the other leg.

Static Quadriceps exercise in lying

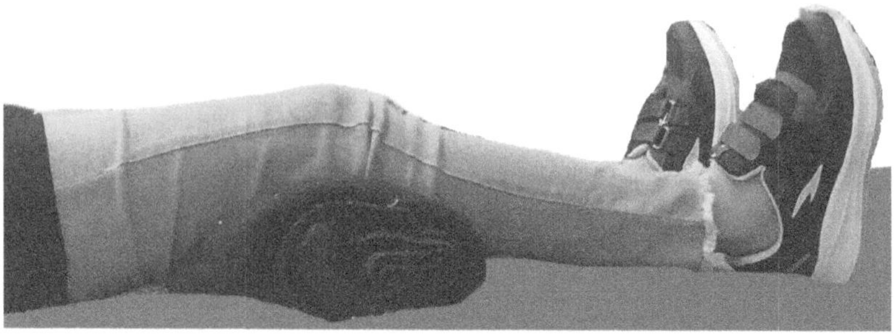

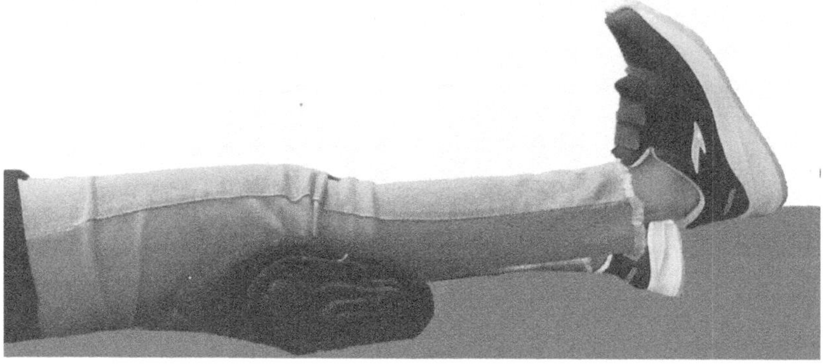

RANGE OF MOTION EXERCISES

Range of motion (ROM) exercises help to improve as well as maintain the flexibility, strength, and function of the knee joint and can help prevent stiffness in the joint.

Some common types of ROM exercises for the knee joint include:

SKATE BOARD EXERCISES:

The individual may use a skateboard or skating shoe to exercise his knee through the flexion and extension, especially during the initial stages of developing knee pain. This helps to a great extent in reducing the inflammation in the knee joint as well as improving the nutrition of the joint cartilage. It is highly advisable for the individual to begin this exercise in the acute stage when he still cannot go ahead with the other simple exercises, such as the static quads. Once he performs these exercises using a skateboard for a few days, he can then slowly transition to the other basic exercises.

Skateboard

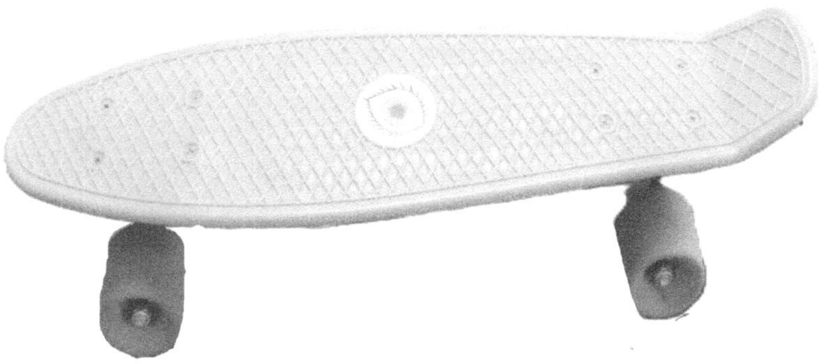

Skateboard exercise (a)

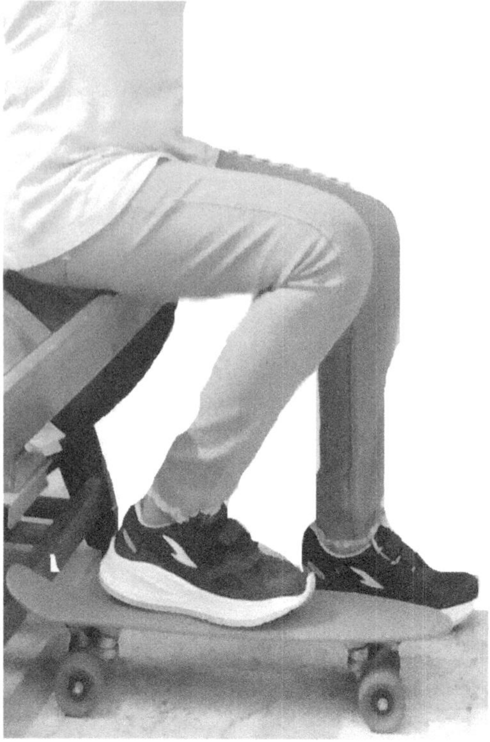

Skateboard exercise (b)

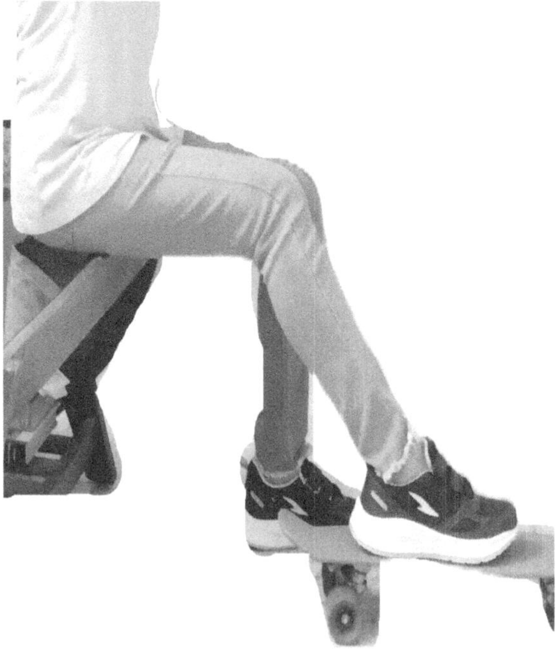

STRAIGHT LEG RAISE:

In this exercise, the individual lies on his back and then slowly raises his leg towards the ceiling with the knee being straight. For those with back pain issues, I would suggest keeping the other knee bent with the foot flat on the floor. This position is maintained for about 15-20 seconds, and then the raised leg is slowly brought back to the initial position. Repeat for several repetitions on each leg.

Straight Leg Raise (a)

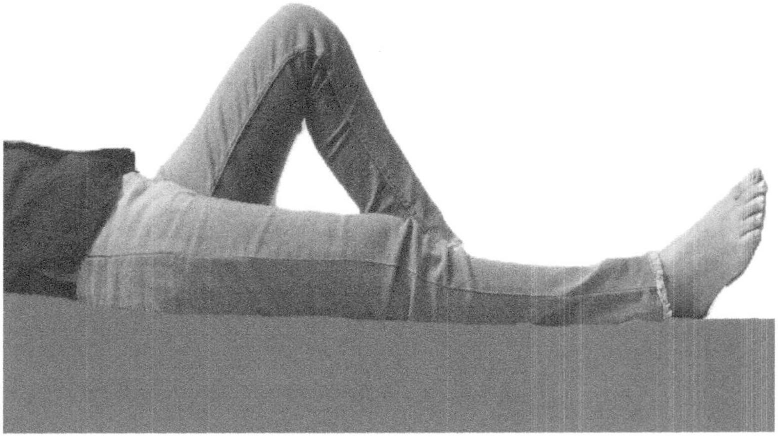

Straight Leg Raise (b)

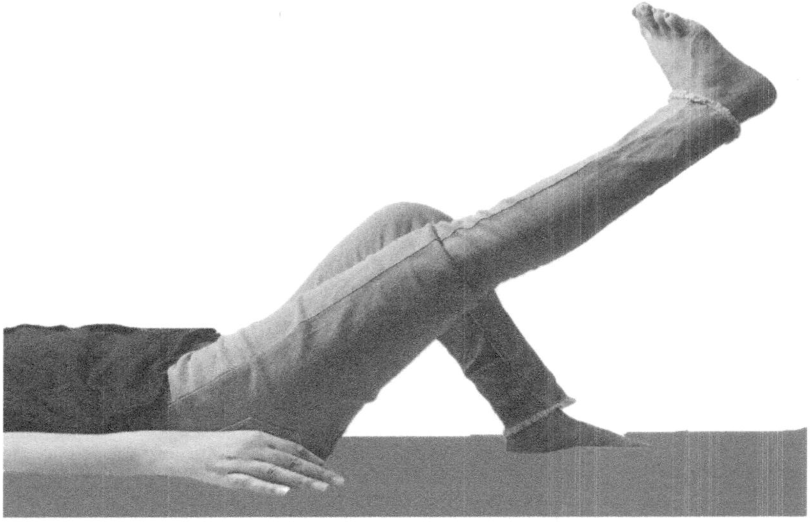

HEEL SLIDES:

The individual lies on his back and then slowly slides one heel towards his hip while keeping the other knee straight. This position is held for a few seconds second, then slowly slide the heel back to the starting position. This exercise is repeated on the other leg.

Heel Slides

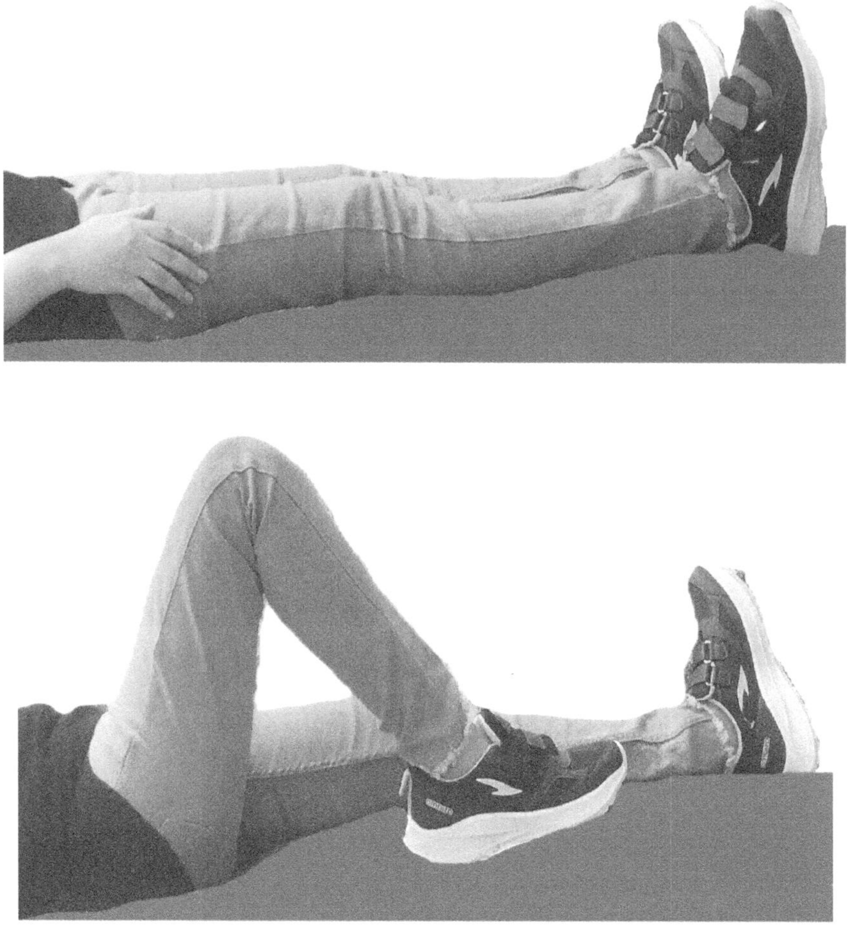

HAMSTRING CURLS:

The individual lies on his stomach and then, thigh, by gently tightening the muscles on the back of the thigh, brings the foot towards the hip. The position is maintained for a few seconds, and then the leg is brought back to the initial position before repeating on the other leg.

Hamstring curls

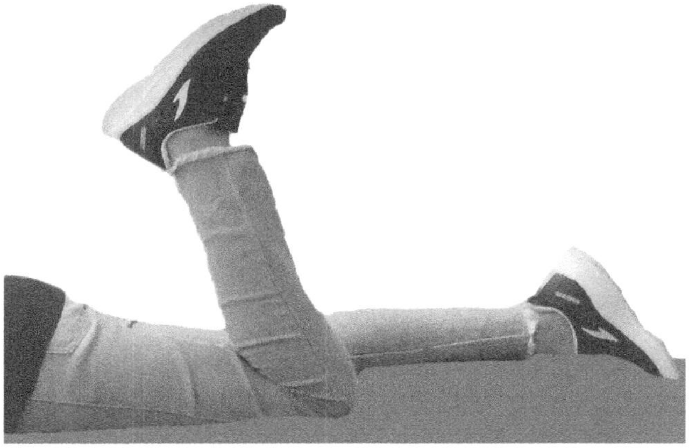

LEG RAISES IN SIDE-LYING:

The individual lies on his side with the lower leg bent towards his trunk as shown in the picture. He then slowly lifts the above limb to around 60 degrees and holds it in this position for about 10 seconds and then gently lowers it back to the starting position. He repeats this exercise ten times for about three sets and then repeats the same on the other lower limb.

Side-lying leg raises

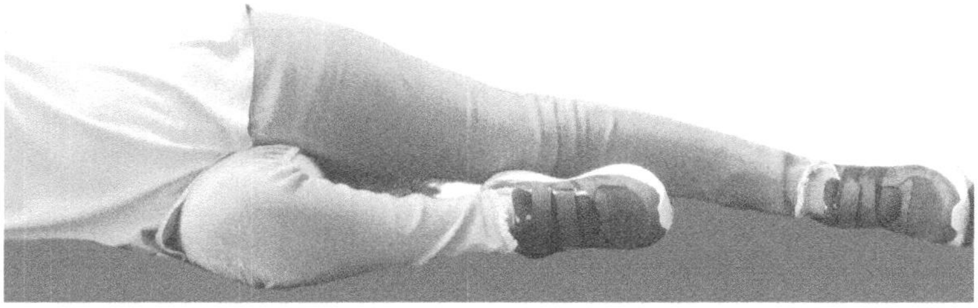

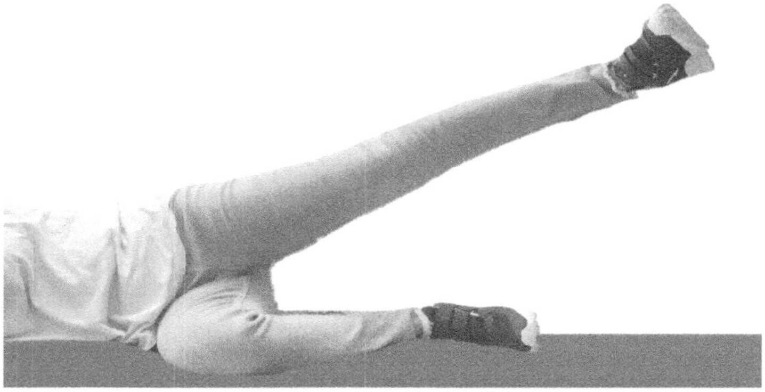

LYING CLAM EXERCISE:

The clam exercise in lying strengthens the muscles around the knee, also improves joint stability, and reduces pain. To perform this exercise, one should lie on his side with his legs bent at a 90-degree angle and feet together. Keeping the feet together, one slowly raises his top knee as high as one can. This position must be maintained for 2-3 seconds, and then the knee slowly lowered back down. This exercise can be repeated 10-15 times for each leg.

Lying clam exercise(a)

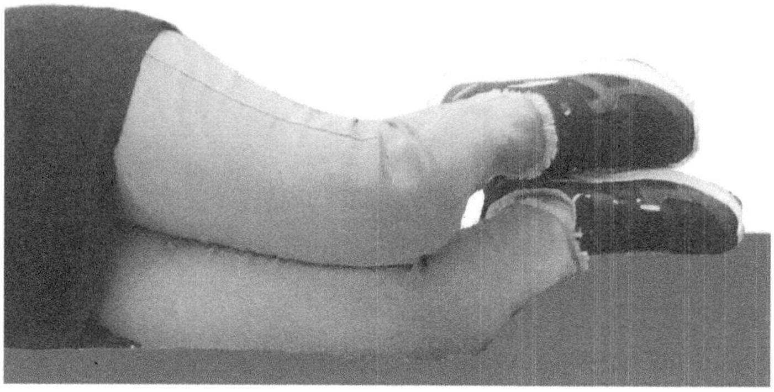

Lying clam exercise(a)

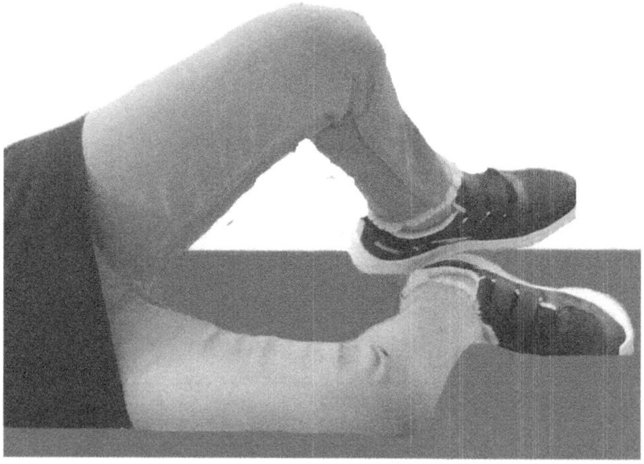

KNEE DISTRACTION EXERCISE WITH ANKLE WEIGHTS:

The individual sits on a high chair or side of the bed with legs freely moving above the ground and with weights around the ankle of the affected leg. He slowly and gently moves his leg forwards and backwards while there is a distraction force applied on his knee due to the ankle weight towards the ground. A small roll of towel can be placed under the thigh for support. The ankle weight can weigh around 1 kg and the exercise can be performed for about 5 to 7 minutes. This exercise technique lacks research and is not evidence based but has been reported to have reduced pain and improved mobility by those who tried this method.

Knee distraction with ankle weight

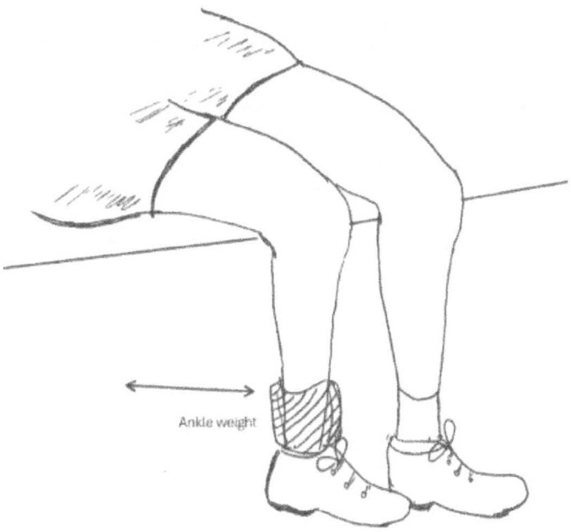

CORE STRENGTHENING

It is important to strengthen the core muscles (trunk muscles) before improving the strength of the lower limb. The core, or the trunk, forms the foundation or base for the movement of the upper and the lower limb muscles. With a weak core, the individual attempting to strengthen the upper or lower limb muscles might be exposed to injuries of the spine. Thus, the trunk muscles, including the back muscles and the abdominals, must be strengthened for one to be truly fit.

STATIC ABDOMINAL EXERCISES:

The individual lies on his back with lower limbs bent as shown in the picture. He may place his hands on his side or across on his chest. He then contracts his belly muscles like tucking in and holding in for about 10 counts. He repeats this exercise about 10 times.

Static abdominal exercise

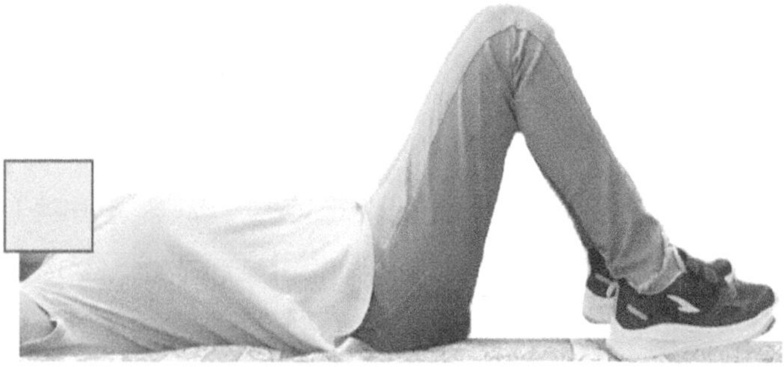

PELVIC BRIDGING:

The individual lies on his back with legs bent. He then tucks in his belly muscles without holding his breath, and then slowly lifts his hip up and holds for about 10 counts. He repeats these exercises about 10 times. This exercise activates the hip extensors.

Pelvic bridging

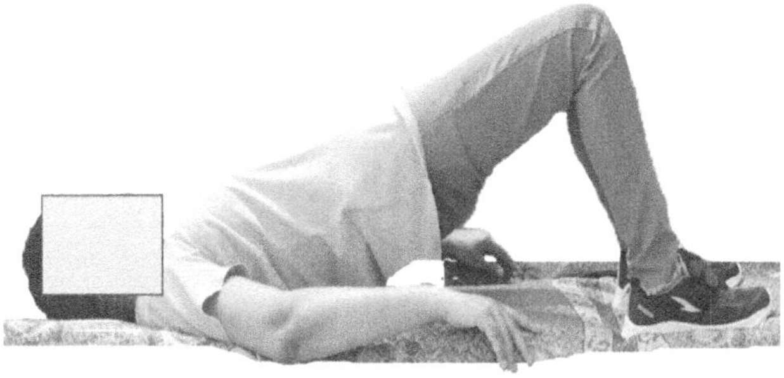

STRENGTHENING EXERCISES

RESISTANCE BAND EXERCISES

Resistance Band exercises, also known as elastic bands, helps to strengthen and stretch muscles. These bands are available in different colours, and each colour has a specific level of resistance. They are used to strengthen the upper body, lower body, and core muscle strengthening, as well as for stretching and gaining flexibility. They also help to improve balance and coordination.

Resistance Band exercises are widely used in rehabilitation post-injuries and post-surgery, as well as to improve general fitness and wellness.

The following are some specific exercises that can be done using a Resistance Band to help with knee arthritis:

STRENGTHENING KNEE EXTENSORS USING RESISTANCE BAND:

This exercise is started with the individual sitting on a chair with the affected knee bent to a 90-degree angle. Then the Resistance Band must be placed around the foot and the ends of the band should be anchored to the furniture behind as shown in the picture. Then the individual slowly straightens the knee, simultaneously pushing against the resistance of the band. After this, the individual slowly returns to the starting position. This exercise is repeated for several repetitions.

Alternatively, the individual lies on his or her chest. One end of the Resistance Band is held with his hands while the other end is placed around the ankle of the affected leg, which is bent at the knee, as shown in the picture. The individual then slowly lowers the leg against the resistance of the band towards the ground. The exercise is repeated several times.

Knee extensor strengthening using Resistance band in lying

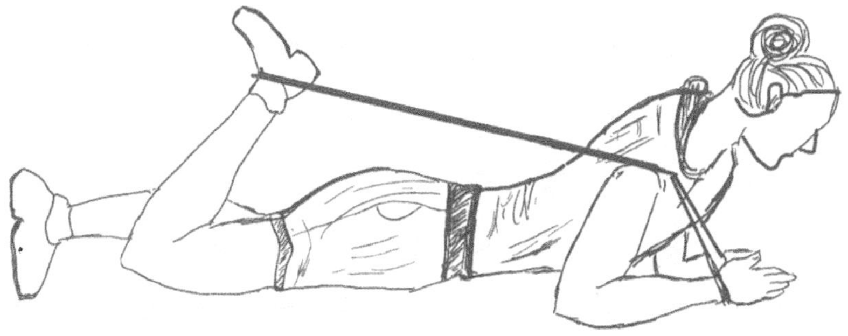

Knee extensor strengthening using Resistance Band in sitting

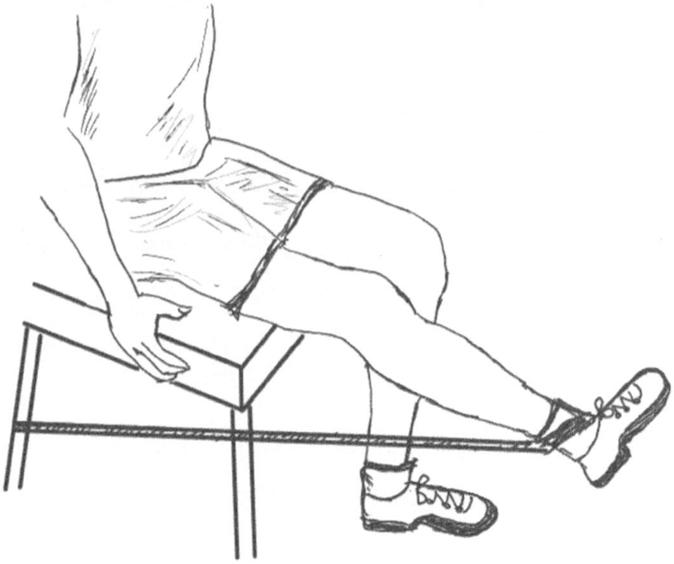

HAMSTRING CURLS USING RESISTANCE BAND:

The individual sits on a chair, keeping the affected knee straight. The Resistance Band is then placed around the foot, with the ends of the band anchored to a furniture in the front. Then the individual slowly bends the knee, pulling the band towards his body. After this, the individual slowly returns to the starting position. This exercise is repeated several times.

Knee flexor strengthening exercise using Resistance Band in standing

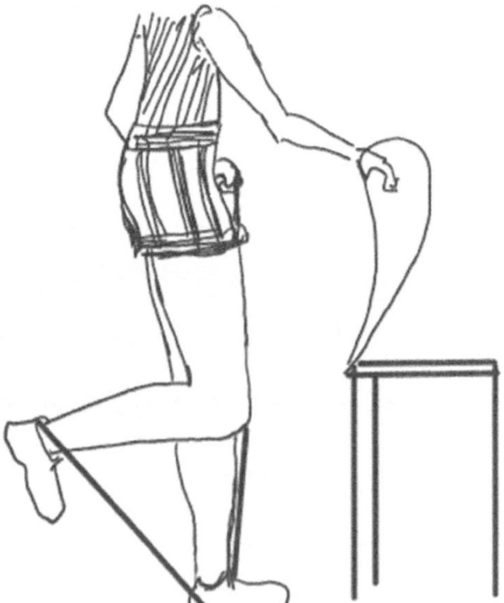

Knee flexor strengthening exercise using Resistance Band in sitting

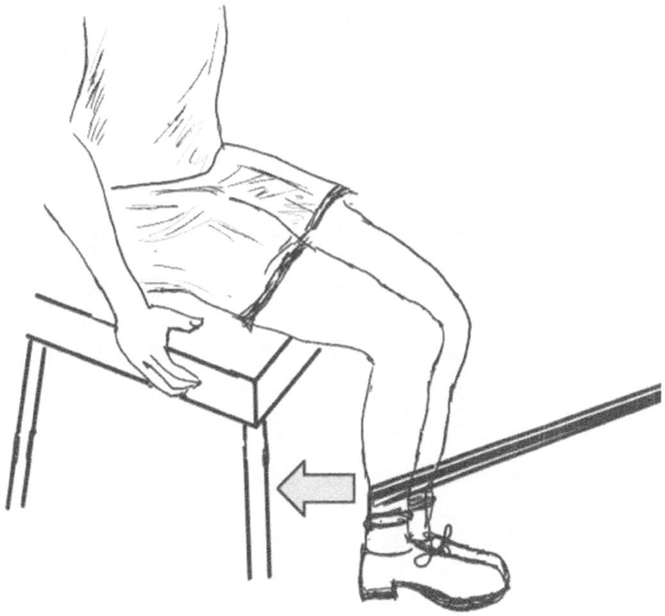

The individual lies on his stomach with one end of the Resistance Band around his ankle and the other end of the Resistance Band anchored to a piece of furniture behind. Then he slowly bends his knee by pulling the heel towards his buttocks. The individual then gets back to the initial position and repeats the exercise several times.

Hamstring curls using Resistance Band

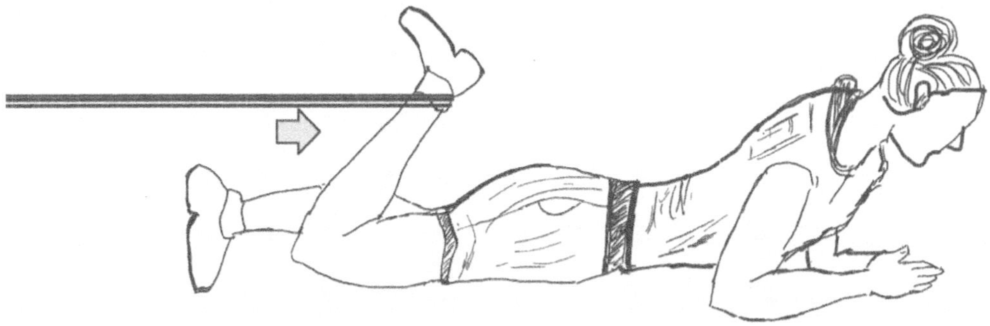

Please make sure to first use a Resistance Band with a low-resistance, and then, as strength improves, slowly progress to higher-resistance resistance bands, or else it might lead to injuries.

HEEL RAISES:

The individual stands with his feet hip-width apart and rises up on his toes. He holds this position for a few seconds and slowly lowers his heels back onto the ground. This exercise helps to strengthen his calf muscles.

Heel raises

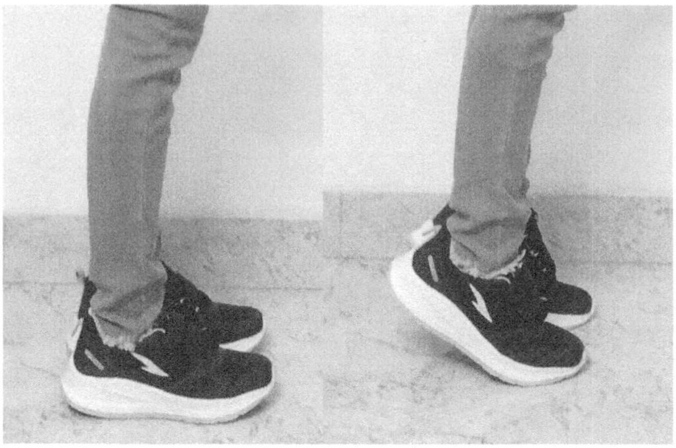

STEP-UPS:

This exercise is beneficial for strengthening quadriceps and hamstrings. The individual stands with a step-in front of him and steps up onto the step with one foot and then gently steps back and down with the same foot and repeats these exercises several times and then performs with the other leg.

Step-ups

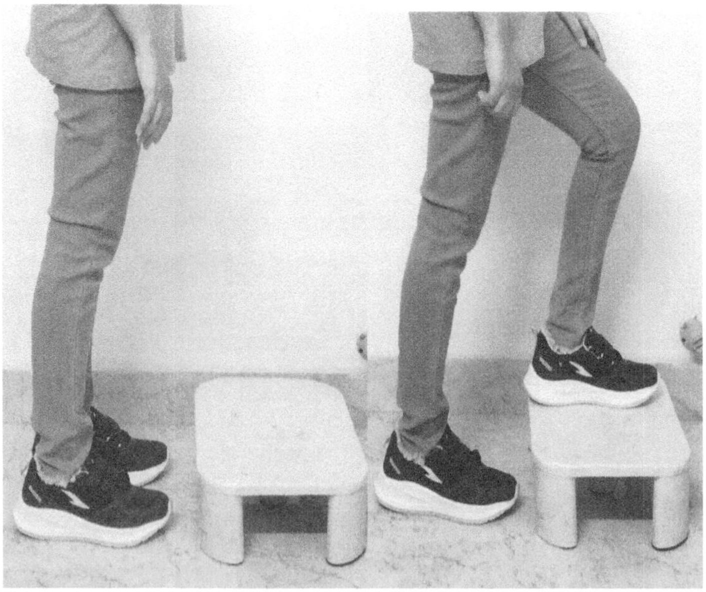

LUNGES:

Lunges help to strengthen the lower limb muscles that include the quadriceps, hamstrings, glutes, and calves. It is a multi-joint exercise that also helps to stretch the hip flexor muscles.

The individual begins this exercise by standing with the feet together. He then takes a step forward with one foot, then lowers the body until the thigh is parallel to the ground, and then pushes back up to the starting position. The process is then repeated several times with the other leg.

CHAIR EXERCISES:

The individual sits at the edge of the chair with his arms crossed. The height of the chair should enable the individual to sit at 120 degrees of hip and knee flexion rather than the 90-degree normal chair. The individual then slightly leans forward slightly, bringing the feet backward, contracting the abdominals as he slowly and gently rises from the chair. He repeats these exercises for another four times to start with and then gradually increases the repetitions to 10 times. Once he masters this exercise, he then repeats the exercises using a chair that allows 90-degree knee and hip flexion.

Chair exercises

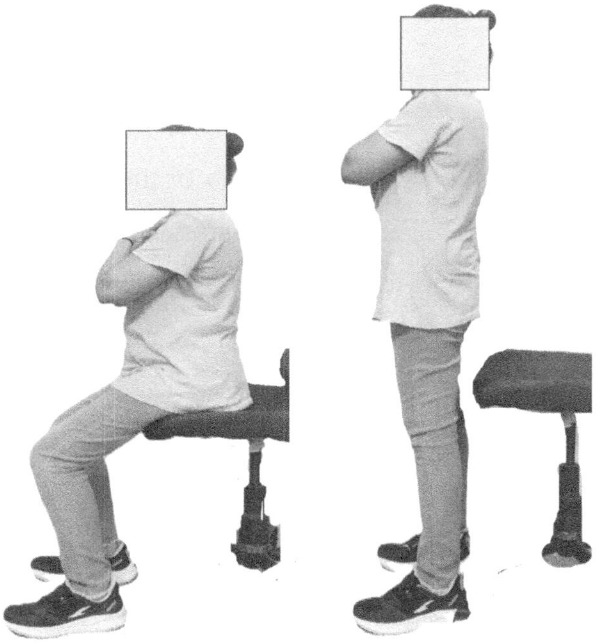

WALL SLIDES:

This exercise is performed with the individual standing with his back against the wall and then slowly sliding down until he reaches a squat position while still keeping his back against the wall. After holding this position for a few seconds, the individual moves back to the original position. This exercise should be avoided if there is any increase in pain or discomfort when performing this exercise after performing these exercises.

Wall slides

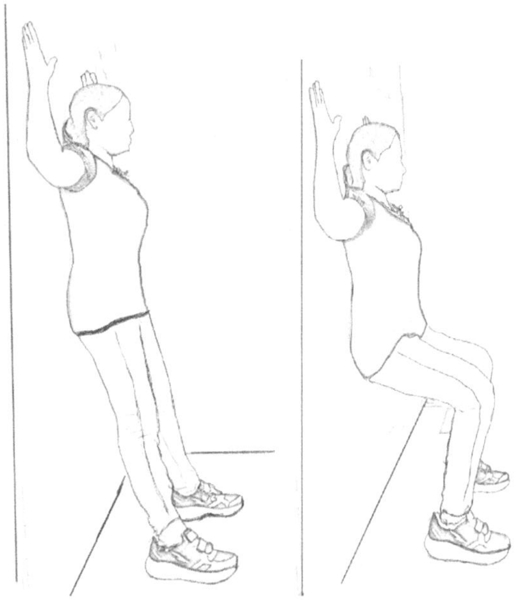

SQUATS:

Squats are beneficial for strengthening the muscles of the lower limb especially the quadriceps, hamstrings and the gluteal muscles. But squats, if started too early in the rehabilitation, may pose greater risk than benefit. It may lead to further cartilage injuries. Therefore, the individual should slowly progress with the exercises in lying, then ROM exercises, strengthening exercises, followed by resistance band exercises and then if comfortable with the knees (without aggravating the existing knee pain) to go ahead with the wall siled and squats.

The individual performs this exercise by standing with his feet apart (shoulder-width) and then slowly lowering his body as if to sit on a chair. His back should always be maintained straight throughout this exercise with his knees behind the toes as one lowers oneself. Holding onto a table or chair could help maintain balance.

SINGLE LEG SQUAT:

This exercise involves the individual bending the unaffected leg at the knee and placing behind on a chair or low table, and slowly bending the weight bearing leg as shown in the picture below. He can take support from a chair or table in the front to avoid fall. These exercises should be performed carefully and attempted only if the individual is capable of doing the squats and other weight bearing exercises such as wall slides and chair exercises (mentioned above) several repetitions without any discomfort or difficulty.

The individual can alternately do these exercises with both feet on the ground as with doing squat and bending his knees slowly with more weight on the exercising leg than the normal leg. This way some of the weight can be offset from the exercising leg thus avoiding overload on the affected knee joint.

Single leg squats

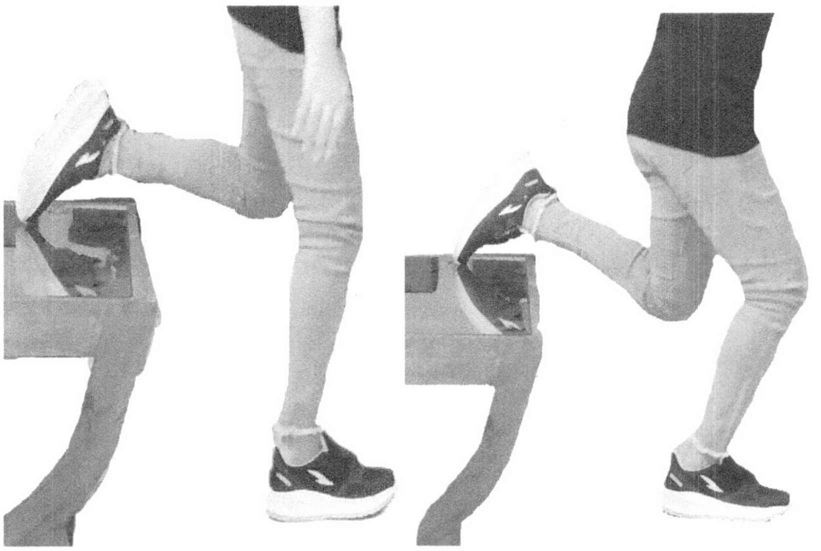

BALANCE EXERCISES:

Balance exercises such as standing on one leg or the wobble board exercises are effective in knee strengthening. They also help to improve the stability of the joint. More about balance exercises will be detailed later in this book.

PATELLAR GLIDES:

Patellar glides are used to improve the function of the knee joint by improving the mobility of the patella in patella-femoral dysfunction. The patient lies in supine with a small towel roll under the knee to maintain the knee joint in slight flexion. Then the therapist applies gentle pressure over the outer border of the patella towards the other knee, thus gliding the patella medially (inwards). The therapist applies gentle pressure over the inner side of patella gently gilding the patella outwards. To glide the patella upwards the therapist applies gentle pressure over the inferior border of the patella and to glide the patella downwards, gentle pressure is applied over the superior border of the patella gliding it in the direction of the foot.

AEROBIC EXERCISES

Aerobic exercise, also known as cardio workouts, is a type of exercise that increases the heart rate and breathing for a sustained period of time. Some examples of aerobic exercise include walking and cycling. Aerobic exercise is an effective way to alleviate symptoms and also improve the overall health of individuals with knee arthritis and cartilage injuries. It is beneficial not only for cardiovascular health but also helps in weight management, improving endurance, lowering blood pressure, and improving cholesterol levels.

The American Heart Association recommends at least 150 minutes of moderate-intensity aerobic activity or 75 minutes of vigorous-intensity aerobic activity per week.

Walking, cycling, and swimming are particularly beneficial for individuals with knee arthritis, as they are low-impact activities that place minimal stress on the joint. Aerobic exercise is beneficial for individuals with cartilage injuries, as it can help to promote blood flow to the affected area, thus aiding in the healing process. By promoting blood flow, it reduces pain and inflammation, thus improving overall joint health and function.

Aerobic exercise can help individuals with degenerative joint conditions to improve their quality of life and stay active. Individuals with cartilage injuries should avoid high-impact activities such as running or jumping, as these can further damage the joint. Instead, they should opt for low-impact activities such as swimming.

Regardless of the type of knee injury or condition, it is important to start aerobic exercise gradually and increase the intensity and duration of the activity over time.

Here are some low-impact aerobic exercises that are good for knee arthritis or those with mild to moderate knee arthritis:

EXERCISE BIKE/STATIONARY BIKE:

This exercise involves sitting on a stationary bike and pedalling with both legs. This is a type of low impact exercise and can help improve the strength, endurance, and flexibility of the knee joint. Cycling helps a great deal in lubricating the joints of the lower limb. Cycling involves pedalling a stationary bicycle.

Cycling is an effective way to improve cardiovascular health and strengthen lower limbs without putting excessive stress on the knee joints and hip joints and is opted for by many individuals who have been having a hard time with arthritis.

SWIMMING: Swimming is a wonderful exercise and has the least impact on the joints. It uses the buoyancy of the water to reduce stress on the joints. Swimming can help improve cardiovascular health and muscle strength without putting stress on the knees. It helps to improve the muscles around the knee joint, improving stability and also reducing pain and inflammation.

WATER AEROBICS: Water aerobics is a great way to improve cardiovascular health and muscle strength without putting stress on the knees. One can stand in the water that is deep enough up to the chest level and walk forwards, backwards, and sideways. This helps in strengthening the muscles of the lower limb. One can also perform forward kicks and also backward standing at the shallow end of the pool. One can also sit on the pool edge and kick the lower legs alternately, which can help in lubricating the knee joints as well as work against the resistance of water to improve muscle strength.

TAI CHI: Tai Chi is considered a low-impact exercise that consists of slow and gentle movements and is helpful not only to improve the muscle tone and strength but also balance and flexibility, a wonderful meditation tool to distract the mind away from the pain.

PROPRIOCEPTIVE TRAINING OF THE KNEE JOINT

Proprioception is the body's ability to sense the position, movement, and tension of muscles, tendons, and joints. Proprioceptive training aims to improve this sense of body awareness and control. The knee joint, in particular, is an important joint for proprioception as it is a weight-bearing joint that is involved in many daily activities such as walking, running, and climbing stairs.

Proprioceptive training for the knee joint typically includes exercises that focus on balance, coordination, and muscle strength. One example of a proprioceptive exercise for the knee joint is the single-leg balance. This exercise involves standing on one leg and holding that position for a certain period of time. The exercise can be made more challenging by closing the eyes or by adding a perturbation, such as a gentle push or pull on the leg.

Another example of proprioceptive training for the knee joint is the mini-squat. In this exercise, the individual stands on one leg and then performs a small squat, making sure to keep the knee joint in alignment with the ankle and hip.

Proprioceptive knee exercises can also be performed with the use of proprioception tools such as a balance board, Bosu ball, or soft foam pad. These tools provide an unstable surface which creates an additional challenge for the knee joint. They can be used to perform exercises such as single-leg balance, mini-squats, and lunges.

Proprioceptive training for the knee joint can also include exercises that focus on muscle strength, such as leg press, leg extension, and leg curl. These exercises help to build muscle strength around the knee joint, which can help to improve knee stability and reduce the risk of knee injury. Exercises such as single-leg balance, mini-squats, and lunges can be performed using proprioception tools These exercises should be done under the guidance of a physical therapist or other qualified healthcare professional.

BALANCE TRAINING FOR THE KNEE JOINT

Maintaining balance in the knee joint is essential for preventing injuries, such as strains and sprains, as well as for promoting overall joint health.

One of the key components of balance training for the knee joint is strengthening the muscles surrounding the joint, including the quadriceps, hamstrings, and calf muscles. These muscles are responsible for stabilising the knee joint and providing support during movement. Strong muscles can help to reduce the risk of injury and improve overall joint health.

Exercises such as squats, lunges, and leg presses can be effective for strengthening the quadriceps and hamstrings, while calf raises can target the calf muscles. It is important to focus on proper form during these exercises to ensure that the muscles are being worked effectively and to prevent injury.

Another important aspect of balance training for the knee joint is flexibility. Tight muscles can put extra stress on the joint, which can lead to injury. Stretching exercises such as hamstring stretches, quad stretches, and calf stretches can help to improve flexibility and reduce tension in the muscles surrounding the knee joint.

In addition to strength and flexibility, balance training for the knee joint should also focus on proprioception, which is the body's ability to sense the position and movement of the joint. Exercises such as single-leg balance, step-ups, and knee stabilisation exercises can help to improve proprioception and promote better balance in the joint.

It is also important to focus on cardiovascular fitness, as a strong cardiovascular system will help to keep the knee joint healthy. Activities such as cycling, swimming, or brisk walking can provide a low-impact workout that is easy on the knees while improving cardiovascular fitness.

TAPING FOR KNEE ARTHRITIS

Taping is a technique that can be used as an adjunct to help alleviate symptoms and improve joint function. The primary goal of taping in knee arthritis is to protect the joint or the part of the body applied to provide support to the joint and the muscles by avoiding stress to the affected area. This can help to reduce pain and inflammation and improve the overall function of the joint and muscles.

The different types or forms of tape include kinesiology tape, athletic tape, and zinc oxide tape.

Kinesiology tape is a type of stretchy, elastic tape that is usually applied to the skin in specific patterns to provide adequate support and thus improve muscle function.

Athletic tape is a stiffer and non-elastic tape that is commonly used to provide support and stability to joints.

Zinc oxide tape is another type of tape used for taping and is strong, adhesive tape used in more severe cases of knee arthritis.

The joint should be clean and dry, and the tape is applied in a specific pattern in order to provide adequate support to the joint and the surrounding muscles. Common tape patterns include the figure-eight pattern, which provides support to the knee joint, and the fan pattern, which helps to support the muscles around the knee.

Taping should not be used as an ongoing solution to knee arthritis and should only be used as a temporary relief or support while other forms of treatment take effect.

MANUAL THERAPY FOR KNEE JOINT

Manual therapy involves the use of hands-on techniques to manipulate the joints and soft tissues of the body. One commonly used manual therapy technique for knee arthritis is joint mobilisation, which involves applying gentle, controlled forces to the knee joint to improve range of motion and decrease pain. Joint mobilisation may help to reduce stiffness and improve the overall function of the knee.

Knee joint mobilisation is a manual therapy technique that can help improve the mobility and function of the knee joint and is performed by a Physical therapist/Manipulation Therapist. It involves the application of a controlled force to the joint in specific directions to improve range of motion, reduce stiffness, and alleviate pain.

Soft tissue mobilization involves massage and other physical techniques to mobilize and manipulate the muscles, tendons, and ligaments that surround the knee joint and thus improve the range of motion and function of the knee joints. Soft tissue mobilisation is beneficial to reduce pain and improve muscle function, which in turn reduces the stress on the knee joint.

Manual therapy is usually a safe and effective treatment option for knee arthritis but is contraindicated in patients with certain medical conditions, such as rheumatoid arthritis, osteoporosis...as it is unsafe and they may not be able to tolerate the forces applied during the procedure.

Manual therapy is commonly performed when there is pain in the movement of the joint, painful bony joint surfaces and soft tissues, and when there is decrease in the joint motion. According to a study published in the journal, Medicina (Kaunas), manual therapy techniques positively contributed in patients with osteoarthritis knee by decreasing the pain and improving function in the joint (Tsokanos A, et al, 2021)

Knee joint mobilisation can be utilised as part of a rehabilitation program and there are several different types of knee joint mobilisation, including:

Gliding: This technique involves gently moving the knee joint back and forth in a smooth, controlled manner. It is used to improve overall joint mobility and reduce stiffness.

Oscillatory: This technique involves small, back-and-forth movements of the knee joint to improve range of motion and reduce pain. It is typically used for patients with knee osteoarthritis.

Distraction: In this technique, a force is applied to the joint in such a way that pulls the joint apart in opposite directions and thus helps reduce the pain and improve mobility. Knee joint distraction has been used in knee osteoarthritis as a joint-preserving technique in order to delay the knee total arthroplasty (Jansen et al., 2020)

Compression: In this technique, a force is applied to the knee joint in such a way that pushes the joint together. There is a joint approximation. Due to cyclic loading of cartilage leading to functional stimulation of the chondrocytes (cartilage cells) and therefore promoting repair of the joint (Noël et al., 2000)

Manipulation: This technique involves a more intense and specific type of force applied on the knee joint. The therapist applies a force that has high velocity but low amplitude and with a short duration and may also involve rotational movement within the anatomical range of the joint. This technique is used to reduce or remove restrictions in the joint (LaPelusa, 2023).

The frequency and duration of knee joint mobilisation will vary depending on the patient's condition and goals. It may be performed as part of a treatment plan that includes other therapies such as exercise, stretching, and use of assistive devices.

Only a trained and licensed practitioner should perform knee joint mobilisation to prevent any further injury due to improper techniques. Patients should be diligent to communicate any discomfort or pain during the treatment procedure.

ELECTROTHERAPY FOR KNEE ARTHRITIS

Electrotherapy makes use of electrical energy in order to heal certain medical conditions. There are several modalities in electrotherapy which can help in pain reduction, improve blood flow to the applied area and promote healing.

There are several different types of electrotherapy that may be used to treat knee arthritis, including:

1. **Transcutaneous Electrical Nerve Stimulation (TENS):** TENS uses low-frequency electrical impulses to help relieve pain and relax muscles by blocking the pain signals from reaching the brain and the spinal cord.

2. **Interferential Therapy (IFT):** IFT uses low-frequency electrical impulses to help increase blood flow and reduce inflammation in the affected joint.

3. **High-Volt Pulsed Current (HVPC):** HVPC uses high-frequency electrical impulses to help promote healing and reduce pain in the affected joint.

4. **Ultrasound Therapy:** Ultrasound therapy uses high-frequency sound waves to help increase blood flow and reduce inflammation in the affected joint.

5. **Laser Therapy:** Laser therapy uses low-level laser light, a beam of light with a specific wavelength, to produce therapeutic effects.

ELECTROTHERAPY MODALITIES FOR KNEE PAIN

TRANSCUTANEOUS ELECTRICAL NERVE STIMULATION (TENS)

TENS is a non-invasive method and involves the application of electrical stimulation by use of surface electrodes to the peripheral nerves. It is used to decrease the pain in an individual (Benoy Benny, 2013).

The duration of TENS treatment for knee arthritis can vary depending on the individual and the severity of their condition. Usually, treatment sessions may last anywhere from 15 to 30 minutes, several times a day. But a study on the duration of TENS application has proved to be effective when applied around 40 minutes per day (Cheing et al., 2003). Some individuals may need daily treatment to manage their symptoms, while others may only need treatment a few times per week.

The settings for TENS treatment will vary and are also specific to each individual. The intensity, frequency, and duration of each electrical impulse can be adjusted. Initially a low intensity is provided, and gradually, as the patient feels comfortable the intensity is then increased.

The frequency of the impulses is typically set between 2 and 150 Hz and the duration between 100 and 300 microseconds. Acute pain is treated with higher frequencies while lower frequencies are used for chronic pain.

The use of TENS is contraindicated in individuals using a pacemaker or other electronic medical device, epilepsy, and pregnancy (Dac Teoli, 2024).

INTERFERENTIAL THERAPY (IFT)

IFT involves the use of two medium-frequency electrical currents that interfere that are applied to the affected area through electrodes. The currents create a therapeutic effect by interfering with pain signals being transmitted to the brain, thereby reducing pain perception.

In general, a typical course of treatment may involve daily sessions for several weeks, with each session lasting between 20 to 30 minutes depending on individual patients' intensity of pain.

The settings for IFT treatment will vary depending on the patient's age, overall health, and the specific type of knee pain they are experiencing. The frequency, intensity, and duration of the electrical stimulation needs to be adjusted to achieve the right outcome.

IFT has been shown to have other beneficial effects for knee pain, such as improving joint mobility and reducing muscle spasms. It is a safe and effective option in managing knee pain.

IFT is contra-indicated in pregnant women, people with heart pacemaker and people with certain skin conditions.

The specific settings for IFT treatment will vary depending on the individual case, but generally, the therapist will start with a low frequency and gradually increase it as the patient becomes more comfortable. The intensity of the electrical impulses will also be adjusted as needed.

The number of sessions and duration of treatment required will depend on the severity of the knee pain and the individual's response to treatment.

HIGH VOLTAGE PULSED CURRENT (HVPC)

HVPC is a form of electrical stimulation therapy that is used to treat a variety of conditions, including knee pain. The treatment settings and duration will vary depending on the specific condition being treated and the individual patient's needs.

For knee pain, HVPC is typically administered using a device that delivers electrical impulses to the affected area. The impulses are delivered at a high voltage and high frequency, which helps to stimulate the muscles and reduce pain.

The treatment settings for HVPC will typically include the amplitude, frequency, and pulse width of the electrical impulses. The amplitude refers to the strength of the electrical impulses, the frequency refers to the number of impulses per second, and the pulse width refers to the duration of each impulse.

The specific settings used for HVPC will depend on the individual patient's needs and the type of knee pain being treated. For example, a patient with chronic knee pain may require higher amplitude and frequency settings than a patient with acute knee pain.

The duration of HVPC treatment will also vary depending on the individual patient and the type of knee pain being treated. In cases of acute pain, a few treatment sessions are sufficient, but in chronic cases, several weeks of treatment may be necessary.

The qualified healthcare professional will determine the best treatment settings and duration based on the individual patient's needs and medical history.

ULTRASOUND THERAPY

Ultrasound therapy is a type of physical therapy that uses high-frequency sound waves to heat the soft tissue in the knee and reduce pain and inflammation. It is commonly used to treat knee pain and arthritis.

The typical settings for ultrasound therapy for knee pain and arthritis include a frequency of 1-3 MHz, a thermal dose of 3-5 W/cm^2, and a duration of 5-10 minutes per treatment area. However, the specific settings used may vary depending on the individual case and the therapist's discretion.

The duration of treatment may vary depending on the severity of the condition and the patient's response to treatment. It may be done as a single treatment or multiple times per week over a period of several weeks.

LASER THERAPY

Laser therapy, which is also known as low-level laser therapy (LLLT) or photo-biomodulation therapy, is a non-invasive treatment modality and involves the use of low-intensity laser beams. It has the ability to stimulate the cells and thereby promote the healing and repair of the damaged tissue. It has been broadly used to control pain and is therefore recommended for its anti-inflammatory effects and efficiency of healing (Youssef EF et al., 2016).

Treatment settings for laser therapy for knee conditions differ depending on the condition of the patient, the specific device, and the protocol that is being used. Typically, a laser with a wavelength between 632 and 904 nm is used, and the energy density (measured in joules per square centimetre) is usually between 3 and 6 J/cm^2 (Youssef EF et al, 2016).

The duration of laser therapy also varies between 2 and 10 minutes per session, and the number of sessions required may depend on the severity of the arthritis and may range from 8 to 20 sessions.

Laser therapy involves the application of the laser beam by directing it at the affected joint through a handheld device, and then the laser energy is absorbed by the cells in the joint, stimulating the production of ATP (Adenosine Triphosphate), the primary source of energy for the cells. This increased production of ATP leads to increased cellular activity and thus helps in the repair of damaged tissue.

Laser therapy has been proved to decrease the pain and inflammation in knee arthritis, and thereby improves the function and mobility in the affected joint (Dompe et al., 2020). Some studies have also suggested that laser therapy may slow the progression of knee arthritis by promoting the regeneration of cartilage (Khumaidi et al., 2022).

ELECTROMAGNETIC FIELD THERAPY (EMFT)

Electromagnetic field therapy (EMFT) makes use of the electromagnetic waves to promote healing and repair the tissues in the body. It is considered a potential treatment for knee arthritis caused by cartilage degeneration, as it may stimulate the growth and regeneration of cartilage cells in the knee joint.

As we age or due to overuse or injury, the cartilage may wear down, leading to pain, stiffness, and decreased mobility and thus decreased function in the knee.

EMFT exposes the affected tissue to the electromagnetic fields, which stimulates the repair and regeneration of cells through a variety of mechanisms that include the activation of the growth factors, the promotion of blood flow to the area exposed, and the stimulation of the immune system.

Pulsed electromagnetic field (PEMF) therapy involves the use of low-frequency electromagnetic waves to create small electrical currents within the cells, which can then stimulate the repair and growth of the cartilage. In a study published in the Physical Therapy' journal, researchers used PEMF therapy on patients with knee osteoarthritis and found that it significantly improved pain and function in the knee (Yang et al., 2020).

Another study, published in the Porto Biomedical Journal, found that PEMF therapy increased the production of proteoglycans (a type of molecule that is important for the structure and function of cartilage) in human cartilage cells in the lab (Andrade et al., 2016). Electrotherapy is promising as a low cost, low-risk and non-invasive techniques that promote healing of the cartilage through the cell-mediated repair (Sakhrani et al., 2022).

Other forms of EMFT that have been studied for knee pain, such as extremely low frequency (ELF) therapy, use electromagnetic fields at a frequency of 50-60 Hz, similar to the frequency of power lines. A study published in the Journal of Rehabilitation Research and Development found that ELF therapy improved pain, function, and quality of life in patients with knee osteoarthritis.

HYDROTHERAPY FOR KNEE ARTHRITIS

Hydrotherapy (also known by different names such as aquatic therapy, water therapy, pool therapy, or balneotherapy) is widely used and uses warmth and the buoyancy of water to support, thus allowing less stress on the joints and muscles. This can be achieved by using a flotation device, such as a buoyancy belt or pool noodle, to support the patient while they perform exercises in water.

The buoyancy of the water helps to take pressure off the joints, thereby reducing the load on the knee joints and thus allowing for a greater range of motion to be regained (Mooventhan & Nivethitha, 2014). The warmth of the water increases blood flow to the area, reduces inflammation, and promotes healing. Hydrotherapy can also improve flexibility and strength to improve the function and endurance of the muscles. This is beneficial in a great way to improve the stability of the joint. Resistance equipment, such as water weights or resistance bands, can be used as a progression while exercising in water.

Hydrotherapy offers an unstable environment and can be used to improve balance and coordination.

Some examples of simple hydrotherapy exercises that can be beneficial for knee arthritis include:

Water walks: Simply walking in the water decreases the load on the knee joint promoting a greater range of motion.

Leg lifts: Lifting the legs up and down in the water can help to strengthen the muscles around the knee.

Knee extensions: Sitting in a chair or bench in the water and extending the knee can help to improve knee strength.

Pool running: Jogging in the water can help to improve cardiovascular fitness and muscle strength.

Balance exercises: Standing on one foot in the water or walking in a straight line can help to improve balance.

Hydrotherapy exercises should be started slowly, and gradually the intensity is increased and the duration of the exercises as one becomes more comfortable and confident in the water. Using the proper technique and form when performing the exercises is important to avoid injury and to maximize the benefits.

Range of motion exercises improve flexibility and mobility in the knee joint, which can be achieved by performing exercises such as knee flexion, knee extension, and leg circles.

Benefits of Aquatic therapy or hydrotherapy for the knee joint:

- Reduced load on the knees
- Reduce inflammation
- Pain relief
- Improved range of motion in the joint
- Faster recovery
- Strengthens muscles

Hydrotherapy may not be suitable for everyone. People with certain medical conditions, such as uncontrolled hypertension or uncontrolled diabetes, and certain skin conditions, such as open wounds or untreated skin infections, should avoid hydrotherapy.

Aquatic Physical therapy has positive effects on the pain, physical activities, muscle strength, and the ability to walk according to a study published in the 'Journal of Orthopaedic Surgery and Research in patients with knee osteoarthritis (Ma et al., 2022)

MYOFASCIAL RELEASE FOR KNEE PAIN

Myofascial release (MFR) is a non-invasive treatment technique used in several musculoskeletal conditions causing pain. It involves the application of a gentle sustained pressure to the myofascial tissues to reduce pain and improve movement and function of the affected joint thus overall quality of life. There are certain points in the myofascia that are pain sensitive, tender points called myofascial trigger points (Lv & that 2024). This is typically done by using the therapist's hands but can also be done with the use of tools such as balls or foam rollers.

The fascia is considered to be a web-like structure surrounding and permeating all muscles, bones, nerves, and organs in the body. It is distributed from head to toe and also plays a significant and crucial role in providing adequate support and protection to all the internal structures. And simultaneously permits movement and flexibility in the body. When the fascia becomes tight or restricted due to the mechanical changes or biomechanical influences such as ageing, hormonal changes, and being overweight, it may cause pain, discomfort, and limited range of motion (Kodama et al., 2023).

There could be imbalances in the muscles and joints that surround the knee joint that can be treated using Myofascial Release (MFR). In the knee, there may be tension in the fascia surrounding the muscles namely the quadriceps, hamstrings, and calf muscles caused by various causes such as overuse, injury, or other chronic health conditions.

Also, there may be tightness occurring in the hip flexors which may in turn lead to the pelvis tilting forward. This may cause indirect straining of the knee joint. This imbalance in the hip flexors can be addressed using MFR, and this correction may thus reduce knee pain.

In a study published in the Journal of Manual and Manipulative Therapy, the participants suffering from osteoarthritis who received MFR were found to have quadriceps, hamstrings, and the calf reported to demonstrate significant improvements in knee pain and knee function. Another study published in the Journal of Athletic Training found that MFR was effective in reducing pain and improving range of motion in individuals with patellofemoral pain syndrome (PFPS), a common cause of anterior knee pain. Participants in the study received MFR to the quadriceps and patellar tendon and reported significant improvements in pain and range of motion after just two weeks of treatment.

A 2017 study published in the Journal of Bodywork and Movement Therapies found that MFR was effective in reducing pain and improving function in individuals with knee osteoarthritis. A 2019 study published in the Journal of Orthopaedic and Sports Physical Therapy found that MFR was effective in reducing pain and improving function in individuals with patellar tendinitis. A systematic review published in the Journal of Bodywork and Movement Therapies also found that MFR was effective in reducing pain and improving function in patients with knee osteoarthritis. The review also analysed the results of 11 studies that included a total of 718 patients. The authors of the review concluded that MFR is a safe and effective treatment for knee osteoarthritis and may be used as an adjunctive treatment to other forms of physical therapy.

Myofascial release is often used in conjunction with other treatments, such as exercise and stretching, to achieve optimal results.

ERGONOMIC SHOES FOR KNEE ARTHRITIS

Wearing proper footwear that provides good support and cushioning helps to decrease stress on the knee joints.

Ergonomic shoes are designed to provide optimal support and comfort for the feet and lower legs, which can be beneficial for individuals with knee arthritis. Some specific features to look for in ergonomic shoes for knee arthritis may include:

- A heel counter that is stable to provide adequate support and stability for the foot
- A cushioned sole to absorb shock and reduce impact on the knee joint
- A firm arch support to redistribute pressure away from the knee
- A toe box wide enough to accommodate and to avoid squeezing the toes thus reducing pressure on the toe joints
- Adjustable straps to accommodate any swelling in the feet and ankle

Ergonomic shoe structure

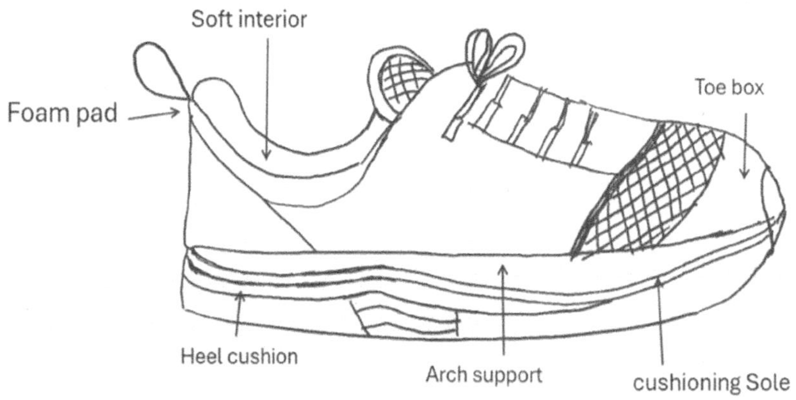

Ergonomic shoes consisting of a rocker sole are helpful to reduce the amount of knee bend (flexion) that is required to push off the ground, allowing walking to be more comfortable and less stressful on the knee joint.

ASSISTIVE DEVICES AND BRACING

The use of assistive devices such as canes and walkers may help reduce the load on the knee joint and improve mobility for people with knee arthritis. Bracing, such as knee sleeves or braces, also provides support to the knee joint and to help reduce pain and inflammation. It is important to ensure that they are appropriate and properly fitted.

KNEE BRACES

There are several different types of knee braces available, each designed to address specific types of knee pain and injuries. These include:

These provide support and stability to the knee joint and can help reduce pain and inflammation. These devices are designed to provide support and stability to the knee joint, helping to reduce pain and improve mobility. Knee braces are available in a variety of styles, including hinged, patella, and neoprene.

In a study published in the Journal of Orthopaedic & Sports Physical Therapy, it was found that knee braces can be effective in reducing pain and improving function in patients with knee osteoarthritis. The study included 132 patients with knee osteoarthritis who were randomised to receive either a knee brace or a sham brace. The results showed that the knee brace group had a significant reduction in pain and an improvement in function compared to the sham brace group (Wang et al., 2007).

A systematic review published in the Journal of Orthopaedic & Sports Physical Therapy found that knee braces are effective in reducing pain and improving function in patients with knee osteoarthritis. The authors concluded that knee braces should be considered as a treatment option for knee osteoarthritis (Brouwer et al., 2012).

Additionally, A case-control study published in the Journal of Bone and Joint Surgery found that knee braces were effective in reducing pain and improving function in patients with knee osteoarthritis when used in combination with physical therapy (Brouwer et al., 2012)

Knee braces offer support to the knee joint, thus reducing the load on the knee joint. They improve the alignment of the knee, reduce pain, and improve mobility.

A type of knee brace, the unloader knee brace, shifts the weight-bearing load away from the affected knee joint and helps reduce the pain and inflammation caused by arthritis. The unloader knee brace is often used for patients with complaints of medial compartment knee osteoarthritis.

The hinged knee brace provides support to the knee joint and prevents excessive movement of the joint. Hinged knee braces are often used for patients with moderate to severe arthritis, as well as for those who have had knee surgery (post-operative management).

Knee Brace

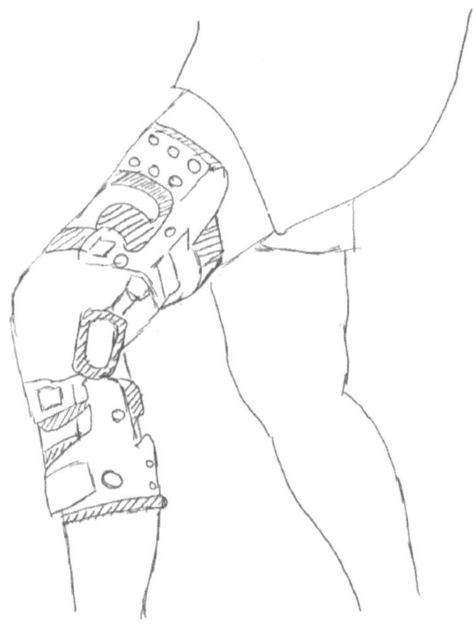

In some cases, a knee brace may not be the most appropriate treatment option, and alternative options such as corticosteroid injections or surgery may be considered.

Additionally, it is important to note that knee braces should be properly fitted and worn as directed by a medical professional. A brace that is not properly fitted can actually worsen symptoms and cause additional pain. It's also important to regularly check the fit of the brace, as the knee can change shape over time due to weight changes or other factors.

KNEE SLEEVE

A knee sleeve is a type of knee support that is worn around the knee to provide compression and warmth to the joint. The compression provided by a knee sleeve can also help to improve blood flow to the knee, which can aid in the healing process. Additionally, the warmth provided by a knee sleeve can help to relax the muscles and joints, which can also help to reduce pain.

Knee sleeve

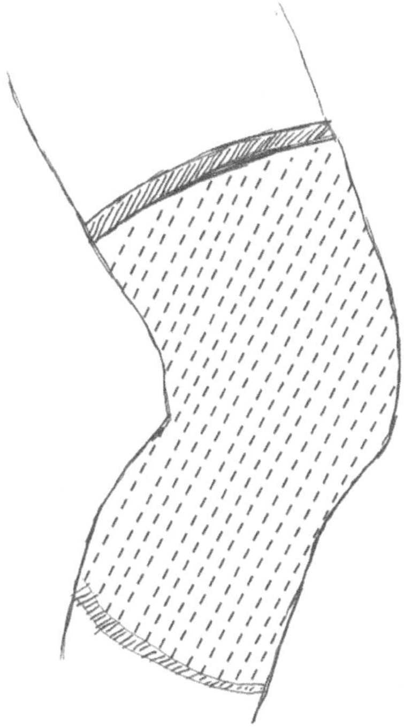

Another study published in the Journal of Rheumatology evaluated the effectiveness of a neoprene knee sleeve in the treatment of knee osteoarthritis. The study included 60 patients with knee osteoarthritis who were randomised to receive either a neoprene knee sleeve or a sham sleeve. The study found that the neoprene knee sleeve group had a significant reduction in pain and an improvement in knee function when compared to the sham sleeve group (Felson et al., 2010).

CANES AND CRUTCHES

Canes and crutches reduce the load on the knee joint and improve mobility and function for people with knee arthritis. They help in redistributing the weight bearing in the joints and thereby decrease the pain and discomfort in the affected knee.

USE OF CANES FOR KNEE ARTHRITIS

Using a cane can be an effective way to manage knee arthritis, as it can help to alleviate pain and improve mobility. However, it is important to use a cane appropriately in order to avoid injury and achieve the maximum benefits.

First, it is important to choose the right type of cane for your needs. There are several different types of canes available, including single-point canes, quad canes, and walkers. Single-point canes have one point of contact with the ground, while quad canes have four points of contact. Walkers, on the other hand, have four legs and provide additional support.

The type of cane that is right for you will depend on your level of mobility and the severity of your knee arthritis. In general, a quad cane or walker is recommended for those with more severe arthritis, while a single-point cane may be sufficient for those with milder symptoms.

When using a cane, it is important to hold it on the opposite side of the affected knee. Canes are typically used with one hand and provide support to the body on the opposite side of the affected knee. For example, if you have arthritis in your right knee, you should hold the cane in your left hand. This will help to take pressure off of the affected knee and improve your balance.

It is also important to use the cane correctly. When walking, lift and place the cane and affected leg forward simultaneously. The cane should be placed on the ground slightly ahead of you, about 12 inches away from the great toe. Then bring the unaffected leg forwards. This will help to take pressure off of the affected knee and improve your balance.

To use a cane safely, you should also make sure that the cane is the right height for you. The top of the cane should reach the level of your hip when you are standing up straight. This will help to ensure that you are using the cane correctly and that it is providing maximum support.

Different types of canes

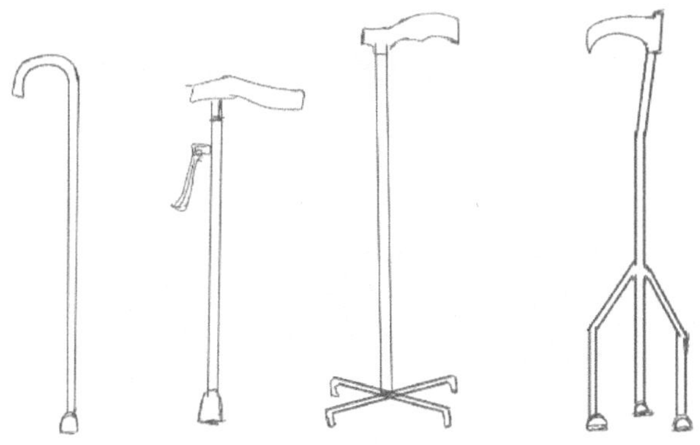

They come in various styles, such as single-point canes, quad canes, and folding canes, and can be adjusted to the appropriate height for the user. According to a study published in the Journal of Orthopaedic Surgery, the use of a cane can reduces the load on the affected knee by up to 25% (Source: "The Effect of a Cane on Knee Load in Patients with Medial Compartment Knee Osteoarthritis" by J Orthop Surg (Hong Kong). 2014 Dec; 22(3): 318–323).

Crutches, on the other hand, are typically used with both hands and provide support to the underarm and hand. They come in different styles, such as axillary crutches and forearm crutches. According to a study published in the Journal of Orthopaedic Surgery and Traumatology, the use of crutches can reduce the load on the affected knee by up to 50% (Source: "Effect of axillary crutches on knee load in patients with medial compartment knee osteoarthritis" by J Orthop Surg Traumatol. 2010 Mar;21(1):11-5)

A Physical therapist can provide instructions on how to properly use the device and adjust it to the appropriate height and ensure that the device is the right one based on the individual's condition.

WALKERS AND ROLLATORS

Walkers and rollators are devices that can be used to assist individuals with knee arthritis in maintaining mobility and independence. Walkers are typically four-legged devices that the user holds onto for support while walking. Rollators, on the other hand, are four-wheeled devices that the user sits on and propels themselves forward with their feet.

To use a walker, the individual should first stand behind the device and grasp the handgrips. The walker should be moved forward in small increments, and the individual should use it for support and balance moving forward. They should take small steps while keeping their hips and trunk aligned over the walker.

Walker

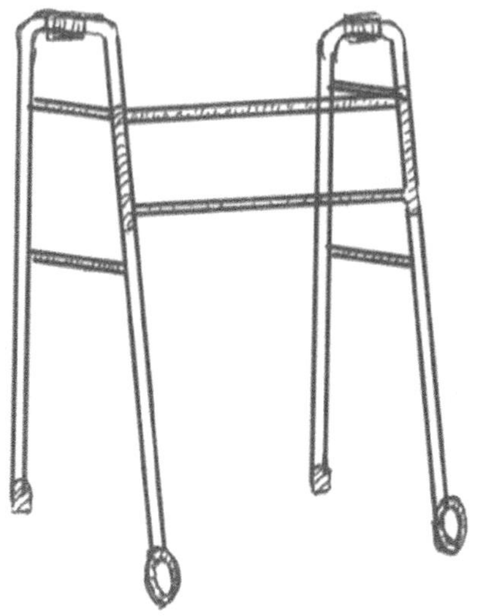

To use a rollator, the individual sits on the seat and grasp the handgrips. They should then propel themselves forward by pushing with their feet. The rollator should be moved in small increments, and the individual should use it for support and balance.

There have been several scientific studies that have investigated the use of walkers and rollators in individuals with knee arthritis. One study, published in the Journal of Geriatric Physical Therapy in 2008, found that using a rollator can improve knee joint stability and gait pattern in individuals with knee osteoarthritis. Another study, published in the Journal of Rehabilitation Research and Development in 2012, found that using a walker can improve functional mobility and reduce pain in individuals with knee osteoarthritis.

HANDRAILS AND GRAB BARS

Handrails can be an effective aid for individuals with knee arthritis to maintain mobility and independence. They provide additional support and stability while walking, which can help to reduce the stress on the knee joint and decrease the risk of falls.

There are several types of handrails that can be used to assist with knee arthritis, including:

1. **Wall-mounted handrails:** These handrails are mounted to a wall and can be used to provide support and stability while walking up or down stairs, or along a corridor and most commonly found in public buildings and homes.

2. **Free-standing handrails:** These handrails are not attached to a wall and can be moved to different locations. They are commonly used in physical therapy settings and can be used to provide support while walking on a flat surface or while performing exercises.

3. **Portable handrails:** These handrails are small and can be easily transported. They can be used to provide support and stability while walking on a flat surface or while performing exercises. They are commonly used by individuals who travel frequently.

GRAB BARS are devices that can be used to provide additional support and stability for individuals with knee arthritis. They can be used in bathrooms, near staircases, and in other areas of the home where additional support may be needed. To use a grab bar, the individual should position themselves close to the grab bar and grasp it firmly with both hands. They should use the grab bar for support and stability while moving in the desired direction. It's important to keep the trunk aligned over the hips and to avoid twisting the spine.

RAMPS AND STAIR LIFTS

Ramps and stairlifts are devices that can be used to assist individuals with knee arthritis in maintaining mobility and independence.

Ramps provide a gentle incline for individuals to walk on, reducing the stress on the knee joint when going up or down stairs. Stairlifts are devices that are attached to the staircases and allow individuals to sit and lift themselves up to the next floor.

To use a ramp, the individual should position themselves at the bottom of the ramp and grasp any handrails that may be present for support. They should then take small steps while keeping their hips and trunk aligned over the ramp. The ramp should be walked up in small increments, and the individual should use it for support and balance.

To use a stairlift, the individual should sit on the seat and grasp the handgrips. They should then press a button or lever to activate the lift, which will then lift them up or down the stairs. The individual should use the handgrips for support and balance while riding on the lift.

When using ramps or stairlifts, it is important to take certain precautions to ensure safety. Ramps should be used on a stable and level surface and should have a non-slip surface. One should always use the handrails or grab bars when available and be cautious when getting on or off the lift or the ramp.

There have been several scientific studies that have investigated the use of ramps and stairlifts in individuals with knee arthritis. One study, published in the Journal of Rehabilitation Research and Development in 2012, found that using a stairlift can improve functional mobility and reduce pain in individuals with knee osteoarthritis.

Another study, published in the Journal of Geriatric Physical Therapy in 2008, found that using a ramp can improve knee joint stability and gait pattern in individuals with knee osteoarthritis.

MEDICATIONS AND TREATMENTS

NONSTEROIDAL ANTI-INFLAMMATORY DRUGS (NSAIDS)

Non-steroidal anti-inflammatory drugs (NSAIDs) are used to treat pain and inflammation. They block the production of certain chemicals in the body that are responsible for inflammation and pain and thus improve function and mobility. Some of the common NSAIDs include Ibuprofen, Naproxen, and Celecoxib.

However, NSAIDs can lead to complications when used long-term or at higher doses. Some potential complications include gastrointestinal bleeding, kidney damage, and an increased risk of heart attack or stroke. Additionally, NSAIDs may be contraindicated in individuals who have certain medical conditions, such as kidney or liver disease, or those who are taking other medications that may interact with them.

Therefore, it is best to use the lowest effective dose for the shortest possible time to minimise the risk of complications under the guidance and as prescribed by the healthcare professional.

STEROID INJECTIONS

Steroid injections are a treatment option for individuals with knee arthritis. They are typically composed of a corticosteroid medication and a local anaesthetic and are used to reduce inflammation and pain in the knee joint. Steroid injections are effective as a short-term treatment option for individuals with knee arthritis, but their effects are typically temporary, lasting for several weeks to a few months (Sihvonen et al., 2017; American Academy of Orthopaedic Surgeons, 2020).

Steroid injections can be used to relieve pain, reduce inflammation, and improve function in individuals with knee arthritis as well as a diagnostic tool, as the relief of symptoms after the injection can help to confirm the diagnosis of knee arthritis.

Overuse of steroid injections can lead to joint damage and can also cause osteoporosis and other side effects and should be used with caution in individuals with diabetes, high blood pressure, or other conditions that may be affected by corticosteroids.

One should be aware of the potential complications and side effects and make sure to not exceed more than three injections per year to reduce the risk of complications.

HYALURONIC ACID INJECTIONS

Hyaluronic acid (HA) injections are another treatment option for knee osteoarthritis and are composed of a naturally occurring substance in the body that plays a key role in lubricating and cushioning joints.

Uses: HA injections are used to alleviate pain and improve function in patients with knee OA who have not responded to other conservative treatments such as physical therapy and oral medications. According to a systematic review by The Cochrane Database of Systematic Reviews, "Hyaluronic acid injections were found to be effective in reducing pain and improving function in people with knee OA" (Cochrane Database of Systematic Reviews, 2015).

Complications: Complications are rare but may include pain and swelling at the injection site and allergic reactions (American Journal of Orthopedics, 2016).

Duration of effect: According to a systematic review by Journal of Orthopaedic Surgery and Research, "The duration of symptom relief varies but generally lasts for 6-12 months" (Journal of Orthopaedic Surgery and Research, 2017). Some studies suggest that repeated injections may provide longer-lasting symptom relief.

The following medications, Disease-Modifying Antirheumatic Drugs (DMARDs) and Biological response modifiers (BRMs) are used in auto-immune related conditions and mentioned here just for information.

DISEASE-MODIFYING ANTIRHEUMATIC DRUGS (DMARDS)

Disease-Modifying Antirheumatic Drugs (DMARDs) are a class of medications that slow the progression of autoimmune arthritis and are commonly used in autoimmune conditions. They are modifying the underlying disease process and can be used in addition to other treatments such as physical therapy and pain management. Some types of DMARDs include methotrexate, leflunomide, sulfasalazine and biologic DMARDs such as TNF inhibitors (etanercept, adalimumab, infliximab) and tocilizumab (Singh, et al., 2015; Smolen, et al., 2016). They prevent joint damage and disability and improve quality of life.

However, DMARDs also have the potential for side effects and require close monitoring by a rheumatologist. They may take several weeks or months before their full effects are noticed, and their potential protocol is individualized. DMARDs may have interactions or contraindications with the other medications being used (Singh et al., 2015; Smolen et al., 2016).

The most common side effects of DMARDs are gastrointestinal upset, infections, and skin reactions. Biologic DMARDs have an increased risk of infections, malignancy, and other side effects and are usually reserved for patients who do not respond to traditional DMARDs (Singh et al., 2015; Smolen et al., 2016).

It's important to follow the guidelines and precautions provided by the rheumatologist or healthcare professional when taking DMARDs. Regular monitoring of liver, kidney, and blood counts is essential, as well as monitoring for infections and malignancy (Singh et al., 2015; Smolen et al., 2016).

BIOLOGIC RESPONSE MODIFIERS (BRMS)

Biological response modifiers (BRMs), also known as biologic DMARDs (disease-modifying antirheumatic drugs), are a separate class of medications and are genetically engineered proteins that work by mimicking the body's own natural defence mechanisms. Some examples of BRMs include TNF inhibitors (Etanercept, Adalimumab, Infliximab) and Interleukin-6 inhibitors (Tocilizumab) (Smolen et al., 2016; Singh et al., 2015). They are effective in treating knee arthritis by reducing pain, inflammation, and joint damage, thus improving physical function and quality of life. They are usually prescribed for patients who have not responded to traditional DMARDs or for patients who have a high disease activity (Smolen et al., 2016; Singh et al., 2015).

As in DMARD's, they may increase the risk of infections and malignancy and may have drug interactions (Smolen et al., 2016; Singh kidney et al., 2015). Regular monitoring of liver, kidney, and blood counts is essential, as well as monitoring for infections and malignancy (Smolen et al., 2016; Singh et al., 2015).

LIFESTYLE CHANGES AND HOME REMEDIES

MAINTAINING A HEALTHY WEIGHT

Weight reduction can help knee arthritis by reducing the amount of weight bearing on the knee joint. When a person is overweight or obese, the extra weight puts more stress on the knee joint, which can lead to inflammation and pain. This is particularly true for people with knee arthritis, as the condition causes damage to the cartilage that cushions the knee joint. The more weight that is bearing down on the joint, the greater the risk of further damage and pain.

According to a study published in Arthritis and Rheumatism (2005), shedding just a single pound of weight can lead to a significant reduction in the load on your knee joints. In fact, the study found that for every pound lost, the load on the knee was reduced by four-fold, making weight loss an effective and a beneficial choice for those looking forward to improve their joint health, particularly given the number of steps we take on a daily basis (Messier et al., 2005)

Weight loss by an individual should be done gradually and in a healthy manner based on the individual's health condition and other comorbidities. Crash dieting or extreme weight loss methods can have negative effects on the body and may even worsen health condition further. A combination of a healthy diet and regular exercise is the best approach to losing weight.

EATING A HEALTHY DIET

A healthy diet is important for managing knee osteoarthritis (OA) and reducing the risk of complications. Some dietary recommendations for knee OA include:

1. Maintaining a healthy weight: As mentioned earlier, obesity is a major risk factor for knee OA, as excessive weight puts extra stress on the joints. Eating a diet that is low in calories and high in nutrient-dense foods can help you maintain a healthy weight.

2. Eating anti-inflammatory foods: Certain foods, such as fruits, vegetables, fish, and nuts, contain anti-inflammatory compounds that can help reduce inflammation in the body.

3. Consuming enough calcium and vitamin D: These nutrients are important for bone health and may help slow the progression of knee OA. Some of the rich sources of calcium include dairy products, leafy green vegetables, and fortified foods. Vitamin D can be found in abundance in fatty fish, eggs, and fortified foods.

4. Limiting processed foods: Processed foods are often high in added sugars, saturated fats, and refined carbohydrates, which can contribute to inflammation and weight gain.

5. Avoiding foods that may trigger inflammation: Some people with knee OA may find that certain foods aggravate their symptoms. Common triggers include gluten, nightshades, and added sugars.

6. Drinking enough water: Adequate hydration is important for joint health and can help reduce stiffness.

It's important to note that a healthy diet will not reverse the degeneration of the joint, but it will help you maintain a healthy weight, reduce inflammation and improve overall health.

ANTI-INFLAMMATORY DIET FOR KNEE ARTHRITIS

An anti-inflammatory diet can be beneficial for individuals with knee arthritis. This type of diet emphasises the consumption of fruits, vegetables, whole grains, lean proteins, and healthy fats while limiting processed foods, sugar, and saturated fats.

According to a study published in the Journal of the Academy of Nutrition and Dietetics, a Mediterranean-style diet, which is rich in anti-inflammatory foods, may improve symptoms of knee osteoarthritis. Another study published in the journal Rheumatology International found that a Mediterranean diet supplemented with extra-virgin olive oil or nuts may reduce the risk of progression of knee osteoarthritis.

Inflammation is a natural response of the body to injury, infection, or other forms of stress. However, when chronic, it can contribute to the development of various diseases such as cancer, diabetes, and heart disease. While there is no single food or nutrient that can completely prevent or cure these conditions, a diet rich in fruits, vegetables, and other anti-inflammatory foods may help reduce the risk of developing these diseases.

Fruits and vegetables are excellent sources of vitamins, minerals, and antioxidants, which have anti-inflammatory properties. Berries, such as blueberries, raspberries, and strawberries, contain high levels of antioxidants, such as anthocyanins, which have been shown to reduce inflammation. Cherries, particularly tart cherries, are also rich in antioxidants and have been found to reduce inflammation and improve symptoms of osteoarthritis. Pineapple contains bromelain, an enzyme that has anti-inflammatory properties and may help reduce pain and swelling.

Tomatoes are rich in lycopene, an antioxidant that has been shown to reduce inflammation and lower the risk of heart disease. Kale, spinach, and broccoli are also rich in antioxidants and anti-inflammatory compounds, such as kaempferol and sulforaphane. Additionally, ginger contains gingerol, a compound with potent anti-inflammatory properties that may help reduce pain and inflammation associated with osteoarthritis and rheumatoid arthritis.

Fatty fish, such as salmon and tuna, are rich in omega-3 fatty acids, which have anti-inflammatory properties. Studies have found that consuming omega-3 fatty acids can reduce inflammation, lower the risk of heart disease, and improve symptoms of rheumatoid arthritis. Olive oil is also a good source of anti-inflammatory compounds, such as oleocanthal, which has been shown to have anti-inflammatory and anti-cancer properties.

Spices like turmeric and garlic also have anti-inflammatory properties. Turmeric contains curcumin, a compound that has been shown to have anti-inflammatory, antioxidant, and anti-cancer properties. Garlic contains allicin, a compound that has been shown to reduce inflammation and lower the risk of heart disease.

It's important to note that the anti-inflammatory effects of these foods may vary depending on the specific compounds and their concentration in the food, as well as an individual's unique physiology and diet. Additionally, consuming a balanced diet rich in fruits and vegetables and limiting intake of processed foods, saturated fats, and added sugars

In conclusion, many fruits and vegetables have anti-inflammatory properties, including berries, cherries, pineapple, tomatoes, kale, spinach, broccoli, and ginger. Other anti-inflammatory foods include fatty fish, such as salmon and tuna, which contain omega-3 fatty acids, and olive oil. Spices like turmeric and garlic also have anti-inflammatory properties. However, more research is needed to understand the specific effects of these foods on inflammation and the mechanisms by which they exert their effects.

QUITTING SMOKING

Smoking is known to have harmful effects on various aspects of health, including in patients with knee arthritis. According to a study published in the journal "Arthritis Care & Research" (Kolasinski, 2019), smoking is associated with increased pain and reduced function in individuals with knee osteoarthritis. Additionally, a meta-analysis published in the "Annals of the Rheumatic Diseases" (O'Neill et al., 2018) found that smoking is a significant risk factor for the development and progression of knee osteoarthritis.

On the other hand, quitting smoking has been shown to have several benefits for patients with knee arthritis. A study published in the "Journal of Rheumatology" (Kong et al., 2016) found that individuals with knee osteoarthritis who quit smoking had improved physical function, reduced pain, and a decreased risk of knee replacement surgery.

In conclusion, smoking has detrimental effects on knee arthritis, whereas quitting smoking has been shown to improve symptoms and decrease the risk of knee replacement surgery.

Smoking is also associated with an increased risk of rheumatoid arthritis (RA), a chronic autoimmune disorder that causes inflammation in the joints and other parts of the body. A study published in the "Annals of the Rheumatic Diseases" (Smoking and rheumatoid arthritis, 2015) found that smoking is a risk factor for the development of RA and that the risk increases with the number of cigarettes smoked and the duration of smoking.

Smoking also negatively impacts the effectiveness of treatment for RA. According to a study published in the "Journal of Rheumatology" (Gladman et al., 2006), smokers with RA had a lower response rate to treatment with disease-modifying antirheumatic drugs (DMARDs) and were more likely to experience disease flares.

REDUCING STRESS

Stress has been shown to have a negative impact on arthritis, particularly in the knee. Stress can cause the release of inflammatory chemicals in the body, which can exacerbate arthritis symptoms such as pain, swelling, and stiffness. Stress management techniques, such as yoga, meditation, and exercise, have been shown to be beneficial in reducing stress and improving symptoms of knee arthritis. Additionally, stress management can also help improve overall well-being, reduce the risk of depression and anxiety, and improve sleep quality.

HERBS AND SUPPLEMENTS

There is some evidence to suggest that certain herbs and supplements may be beneficial for managing knee arthritis symptoms. Extensive research is needed to confirm their effectiveness, and they should not be used as a substitute for conventional medical treatment.

- **Glucosamine and chondroitin sulphate**, the two health supplements, are compounds that are found naturally in cartilage and may help decrease the inflammation and improve joint function. A meta-analysis of trials published in the journal "Osteoarthritis and Cartilage" in 2010 found that the combination of glucosamine and chondroitin sulphate may be effective in reducing pain and improving physical function in knee osteoarthritis (Bruyère et al., 2010).

- **Boswellia (Indian frankincense)** is a herb that is known to have anti-inflammatory properties. A study published in the journal "Phytotherapy Research" in 2012 found the effectiveness of Boswellia in reducing knee pain and improving function in people suffering with osteoarthritis (Gupta et al., 2012).

- **Curcumin** is a compound found in turmeric and is known for its anti-inflammatory and antioxidant properties. A randomised controlled trial published in the journal "Phytotherapy Research" in 2012 found that curcumin was effective in reducing pain and improving function in people with knee osteoarthritis (Belcaro et al., 2012).

COPING WITH THE EMOTIONAL IMPACT OF KNEE ARTHRITIS

UNDERSTANDING THE EMOTIONAL EFFECTS OF CHRONIC PAIN

Chronic pain can have a significant effect on a person's emotions. It may have a wide range of effects, such as sleep disturbances, fatigue, irritability, and poor concentration, and may further exacerbate emotional symptoms. Chronic pain may cause frustration, as it will be difficult for people to enjoy their daily lives and reduce their efficiency to be productive, making them angry.

People may feel uncertain about the pain getting worse and their inability to manage pain, causing anxiety leading to nervousness and agitation. People may feel hopeless, helpless, and despairing. They may not be able to relax. Their socialisation may be affected by their feelings of isolation and loneliness.

People can manage their pain effectively and avoid the emotional impact of pain by simply choosing to be in the present. Being in the present, practiced widely all over the world, is that state of awareness when one is engaged in the present moment without judging or being distracted.

STRESS MANAGEMENT TECHNIQUES

Some of the effective ways to be in the present are as follows:

Meditation: Meditation may include focused breathing exercises, guided meditations, mindfulness or simply sitting quietly and observing one's thoughts without engaging with them.
Yoga or other movement practices: Engaging in physical activities such as yoga, tai chi, or qigong may also help bring one to be in the present moment by focusing on one's breath and movements.

Nature: Spending time in nature and connecting with the natural world can help to focus on the present moment and let go of distractions and may help to reduce stress and anxiety and promote feelings of peace and tranquillity.

Journaling: Reflecting on the present moment and writing down one's thoughts and feelings can help one to focus on the present and understand their thoughts better.

Mindful eating: One way to be present is to slow down while eating and savour one's food. Paying attention to the taste, smell, and texture of the food, and avoiding distractions like TV or phone while eating.

Engage with your senses: Focus on what you can see, hear, feel, smell, and taste in the present moment. This can help one to be more aware of their surroundings and the present moment.

Be kind to yourself: Accept the present moment as it is, without judgement. This can help you to let go of thoughts of the past or future and focus on the present.

Progressive muscle relaxation: This technique involves tensing and then relaxing different muscle groups to release tension and promote relaxation.

Diaphragmatic breathing: This involves taking deep breaths from the diaphragm, which can help calm the mind and reduce stress.

Gratitude practice: Taking time to reflect on things you are grateful for can help shift your focus to the present moment and away from worries about the past or future.

It's important to note that what works for one person may not work for another, so it's good to try different techniques and find what works best for you.

Being in the present moment is a skill that requires practice and patience. With time, you'll find it easier to be in the present moment and enjoy the many benefits it can bring, such as reducing stress and increasing overall well-being.

MINDFULNESS TO DEAL WITH CHRONIC PAIN

Mindfulness is a form of meditation in which an individual focuses their attention on the present moment without judgement. Mindfulness has recently gained attention all over the world as a simple yet effective means of being in the present. It has been found to be effective in reducing chronic pain.

Mindfulness techniques can help individuals learn to accept and cope with their pain, rather than constantly struggling against it. Mindfulness has been shown to help with chronic pain by altering the way the brain processes the pain. Research has found that mindfulness practices can alter activity in the brain regions involved in pain perception, resulting in a reduction in pain.

To practice mindfulness for chronic pain, individuals can try a variety of techniques such as:

- **Body scan:** This involves lying down and systematically focusing on each part of the body, noting any sensations of pain or discomfort.

- **Breathing exercises:** Focusing on the breath can help an individual stay present and calm and can also help to reduce muscle tension, which can exacerbate pain.

- **Guided imagery:** Sitting quietly in a calm place and visualizing a peaceful scene may help to reduce stress and pain.

- **Yoga:** Yoga combines movement, breath, and meditation, which can help to increase flexibility and reduce pain.

- **Mindful movement**, such as Tai Chi or Qi Gong, can help to reduce pain by improving balance and posture.

Overall, mindfulness can be a powerful tool for managing chronic pain. With regular practice, mindfulness can help individuals learn to live with chronic pain in a more manageable way.

EMOTIONAL FREEDOM TECHNIQUE FOR KNEE PAIN

Emotional Freedom Technique (EFT) is a form of psychological acupressure that involves tapping on specific acupoints on the body while focusing on a specific emotional or physical issue. The technique is based on the idea that negative emotions and physical pain are the result of disruptions in the body's energy system and that tapping on these acupoints can help to restore balance and alleviate symptoms.

In the case of knee arthritis, EFT can be used to address both the physical pain associated with the condition and any emotional or psychological distress that may be exacerbating the pain.

To begin an EFT session for knee arthritis, the individual would first identify the specific issue or problem they wish to address. This could include the physical pain in their knee, as well as any emotional or psychological factors that may be contributing to the pain, such as anxiety or stress.

Next, the individual would tap on specific acupoints on the body while focusing on the issue at hand. These acupoints include the top of the head, the eyebrows, the side of the eyes, the under the eyes, under the nose, under the lips, collarbone, under the arm, and the wrist.

As the individual taps on each acupoint, they would repeat a specific phrase, such as "Even though I have this pain in my knee, I deeply and completely accept myself." This phrase is known as a "setup statement" and is intended to help the individual focus on the issue at hand and release any negative emotions or thoughts that may be contributing to the pain.

After tapping on each acupoint, the individual would then take a deep breath and assess any changes in the intensity of their pain. If the pain has not decreased significantly, the individual may repeat the process several more times.

However, it is important to note that EFT should not be used as a substitute for traditional medical treatment and should always be used in conjunction with a healthcare provider.

Here is an example of how EFT can be used for knee arthritis:

1. The issue is identified and, in this book, since we are discussing about managing knee arthritis, we shall consider the issue of knee arthritis and the discomfort that it causes
2. Rating the intensity of pain and discomfort on a scale of 0-10
3. Setting up a statement is setting up a phrase that will acknowledge the current issue (knee arthritis pain and discomfort) and also to include a reminder to be open to the healing process. For example: " Even though I have this pain and discomfort in my knee from my arthritis, I deeply and completely accept myself."
4. Tapping on the points mentioned below while repeating the set-up statement:

- The top of your head
- Your inner eyebrow
- The side of your eye
- Under your eye
- Under your nose
- On your chin

- On the collarbone
- Under your arm
- On your wrist

5. **Re-assessment:** The individual then re-assesses the intensity of pain and his discomfort after tapping for a few minutes. Most likely it would have been comparatively decreased
6. The individual then repeats this process until he feels the pain and discomfort has reached a manageable level.

Studies have shown that EFT can reduce pain, improve physical function, and reduce the need for pain medication in people with knee arthritis.

FINDING SUPPORT FROM FAMILY AND FRIENDS

Finding support from family and friends can be an important part of managing the condition and maintaining a good quality of life. Here are some ways that family and friends can support someone with arthritis:

Understanding the condition: The caretakers, family, and friends of the patient can educate themselves about arthritis and how arthritis can affect the patient so that they can understand the challenges the patient faces and help them in the best possible way.

Help with daily tasks: People with arthritis may have difficulty with certain tasks, such as cooking, cleaning, or dressing. Offering to help with these tasks can be a big help and can make a huge difference in the person's day-to-day life.

Encourage exercise: Regular exercise is an important part of managing arthritis. Encouraging the patient to engage in regular physical activity, such as walking or swimming, can help them to maintain mobility and reduce pain.

Listen and be understanding: People with arthritis may experience emotional ups and downs related to the condition. Being a listening ear and being understanding when the person talks about their feelings can be very important.

Accompany to medical appointments: Going to medical appointments can be overwhelming; having a family member or friend to accompany the person to their appointments can provide emotional support and help them understand their condition better.

Help with transportation: Arthritis can make it difficult to drive or use public transportation. Offering to drive the person to appointments or errands can be a big help.

Encourage social activities: People with arthritis may be hesitant to participate in social activities because of the pain or fatigue caused by their condition. Encouraging the person to participate in social activities can help them to maintain a good quality of life and prevent feelings of isolation.

By providing practical and emotional support, family and friends can help the person with arthritis to maintain a good quality of life and manage the challenges of the condition.

PROGNOSIS AND POTENTIAL COMPLICATIONS OF KNEE ARTHRITIS

Knee arthritis is a chronic condition that can affect an individual's quality of life in a significant way. The prognosis of knee arthritis varies depending on the type of arthritis, the severity of symptoms of the affected joint or joints, and the individual's overall health.

The symptoms of knee arthritis can vary from person to person and may change over time as the condition of the affected joint progresses. Some people may have mild symptoms while others may have severe symptoms.

Osteoarthritis, as mentioned earlier, typically worsens over time. As the condition progresses, the joint may become increasingly deformed, and the cartilage may continue to wear away. (American Academy of Orthopaedic Surgeons, 2021) This can lead to chronic pain, stiffness, and difficulty with performing daily activities. In advanced cases of arthritis, joint replacement surgery may be required to improve function, alleviate pain, and thus improve the quality of life. Osteoarthritis in later stages may lead to the formation of bony spurs that may cause irritation of the joint and its surrounding structures, falling leading to an increase in pain. Patients with osteoarthritis have an increased risk of fall due to weakness and instability at the affected joint.

Rheumatoid arthritis is an autoimmune condition that can also affect the knee joint. Rheumatoid arthritis may lead to deformed joints and erosion of the bones. (Arthritis Foundation, 2021) This can affect the quality of life in a significant way as the activities of daily life become painful. With proper treatment for the condition, such as disease-modifying antirheumatic drugs (DMARDs) and biologic agents, the progression of the disease can be slowed, and joint damage can be further delayed or prevented.

Post-traumatic arthritis can cause painful, stiff and deformed joints if right care at the right time not given (OrthoInfo, 2021)

It is important to note that the prognosis and potential complications of knee arthritis can vary from person to person and may change over time as the condition progresses.

In addition, knee arthritis can lead to decreased physical activity and a decrease in overall physical fitness, which can lead to other health problems such as obesity, diabetes, and heart disease. According to a study by the National Centre for Biotechnology Information, "physical therapy and exercise can improve pain and function in individuals with knee osteoarthritis." (Gustafson, Roos, Lohmander & Ljungberg, 2004)

Surgery can also be an option for individuals with knee arthritis, particularly for those with advanced osteoarthritis or post-traumatic arthritis. According to the American Academy of Orthopaedic Surgeons, "joint replacement surgery can significantly improve function and alleviate pain in individuals with knee osteoarthritis." (American Academy of Orthopaedic Surgeons, 2021.

PLANNING FOR THE FUTURE: SURGERY AND OTHER OPTIONS

SURGICAL MEASURES FOR CARTILAGE INJURIES

In cases of severe or serious cartilage injuries, several surgical procedures are available depending on the type and severity of injury. The commonly used surgical procedures include microfracture, osteochondral autograft transfer system (OATS), autologous chondrocyte implantation (ACI), and autologous matrix-induced chondrogenesis (AMIC).

Now let's discuss each of the procedures in more detail. Microfracture is a procedure in which small holes are made in the bone to encourage the growth of new cartilage. OATS is a procedure in which a small piece of healthy cartilage is taken from another part of the knee and used to replace the damaged cartilage. ACI and AMIC are the procedures where a small piece of cartilage is taken from the patient's own knee joint and then grown in a lab before long-term transplantation back into the patient's knee.

WHEN TO CONSIDER SURGERY

Surgery is typically considered for patients with knee arthritis as a last resort, after other treatments such as physical therapy, weight loss, and medication have failed to provide sufficient relief.

A systematic review published in the Journal of Bone and Joint Surgery in 2014 found that "nonoperative management should be the first-line treatment for most patients with knee osteoarthritis" (Koch, 2014).

A clinical practice guideline from the American Academy of Orthopaedic Surgeons (AAOS) states that "surgery should be considered only after a trial of nonoperative management has failed to provide adequate pain relief and improvement in function" (AAOS, 2013).

A study published in the Journal of the American Medical Association in 2012 found that "physical therapy and exercise were more effective than arthroscopy in reducing pain and improving function in patients with knee osteoarthritis" (Losina, 2012).

Criteria for surgery in patients with knee arthritis typically include:

- Failure of non-surgical treatment options such as physical therapy, weight loss, and medication to provide adequate pain relief and improvement in function.
- Presence of specific structural abnormalities, such as a large joint effusion or osteophytes, that can be addressed surgically.
- Quality of life significantly impacted by the knee arthritis.

TYPES OF KNEE SURGERIES

Surgical options for knee arthritis include:

Arthroscopy: It is a procedure that uses a small camera to look inside the joint and remove or repair damaged tissue. A study published in The Journal of Bone and Joint Surgery in 2016 found that "Arthroscopy for the treatment of knee osteoarthritis is not recommended in patients with mild or moderate disease." (Mink, 2016)

Osteotomy: The procedure involves cutting and reshaping the bone to realign the joint and redistribute weight-bearing forces. A systematic review published in the Journal of Bone and Joint Surgery in 2014 found that "osteotomy may be considered in selected patients with medial compartment knee osteoarthritis, particularly those with varus alignment, a young age, and good bone stock" (Koch, 2014).

Arthroplasty: This is the replacement of the damaged joint surfaces with an artificial implant, which can be either a total knee replacement or a partial knee replacement. A study published in the Journal of Arthroplasty in 2017 found that "Total knee arthroplasty (TKA) is considered as a gold standard for end-stage knee osteoarthritis is (KOA)." (Kwok, 2017).

ARTHROSCOPIC SURGERIES FOR KNEE CARTILAGE

Arthroscopy is a surgical procedure that allows doctors to look inside a joint using a small camera called an arthroscope. This procedure is commonly used to diagnose and treat problems in the knee, but it can also be used on other joints such as the shoulder, elbow, ankle, and wrist.

During a knee arthroscopy, a small incision is made in the skin, and the arthroscope is inserted into the joint. The camera at the end of the arthroscope sends images of the inside of the joint to a monitor, allowing the doctor to see the condition of the knee cartilage, ligaments, and other structures.

One of the most common reasons for knee arthroscopy is to repair or remove the damaged cartilage. Arthroscopy is used to remove small pieces of loose cartilage or to smooth out rough edges of cartilage. In some cases, the doctors may use a technique called microfracture that can stimulate the growth of new cartilage. This is done by making small holes in the bone to encourage the growth of new cartilage.

Another common reason for knee arthroscopy is to repair or reconstruct torn ligaments. The knee has four ligaments that provide stability and support: the anterior cruciate ligament (ACL), posterior cruciate ligament (PCL), medial collateral ligament (MCL), and lateral collateral ligament (LCL).

During a knee arthroscopy, the doctor can repair or reconstruct a torn ligament using sutures, screws, or other devices. This can help to restore stability to the knee and reduce pain and swelling.

Arthroscopy is generally considered a safe and effective procedure, with a high success rate. The most common risks associated with knee arthroscopy include infection, bleeding, and reactions to anaesthesia. In rare cases, there may be nerve or blood vessel injury, or the procedure may not be successful in resolving the patient's pain or restoring the joint's function.

Recovery time can vary depending on the individual's type of procedure and the patient's overall health and comorbidities. Most people are able to return to normal activities within a few weeks to a few months. Physical therapy may be required to help regain strength and mobility in the knee.

POTENTIAL RISKS AND BENEFITS

The potential risks and benefits of surgical options for knee arthritis include:

Arthroscopy:

- **Benefits:** can provide pain relief in patients with mild to moderate knee osteoarthritis and some improvement in function.
- **Risks:** Risks include infection, bleeding, and complications related to anaesthesia. A study published in The Journal of Bone and Joint Surgery in 2016 found that "Arthroscopy for the treatment of knee osteoarthritis is not recommended in patients with mild or moderate (Mink, 2016).

Osteotomy:

○ **Benefits:** Can provide significant pain relief and improvement in function for patients with specific structural abnormalities, such as a large joint effusion or osteophytes, and good bone stock.

○ **Risks:** May require a longer recovery period and a risk of implant failure or other complications. A systematic review published in the Journal of Bone and Joint Surgery in 2014 found that "osteotomy may be considered in selected patients with medial compartment knee osteoarthritis, particularly those with varus alignment, a young age, and good bone stock" (Koch, 2014).

Arthroplasty:

○ **Benefits:** Can provide significant pain relief and improvement in function for patients with end-stage knee arthritis and can improve the quality of life.

○ **Risks:** Long-term risks include implant failure, infection, and blood clots, as well as the need for revision surgery. A study published in the Journal of Arthroplasty in 2017 found that "Total knee arthroplasty (TKA) is considered as a gold standard for end-stage knee osteoarthritis (KOA), but it is associated with some risks such as infection, blood clots, and implant failure" (Kwok, 2017).

REHABILITATION AND RECOVERY

Rehabilitation and recovery after surgical treatment for knee arthritis is an important aspect of the overall treatment process. The specific rehabilitation protocol will vary depending on the type of surgery performed and the individual needs of the patient. However, there are some general principles that are commonly followed for patients who have undergone surgery for knee arthritis.

Rehabilitation should be started as soon as possible after the surgery. This can be simple exercises to start with, such as range of motion exercises, such as flexion and extension exercises, as well as exercises to strengthen the muscles around the knee, the quadriceps, hamstrings, and calf muscles.

Physical therapy is an important part of postoperative rehabilitation. A physical therapist will work with the patient to help them regain their strength, flexibility, and range of motion. They will also teach the patient exercises that will help them maintain their progress and prevent further injury. Physical therapy sessions can include a combination of exercises, manual therapy techniques, and modalities such as ultrasound, electrical stimulation, and ice or heat. A study published in the Journal of Orthopaedic Surgery and Research in 2016 found that "Physical therapy and exercise are essential components of postoperative rehabilitation for patients who have undergone knee arthroplasty" (Liu, 2016)

A study published in the Journal of Arthroplasty in 2015 found that "patients who undergo total knee arthroplasty require a structured rehabilitation program to achieve optimal functional outcomes." (Ritter, 2015). Patients will also be instructed on the use of crutches, walkers, or canes, as well as how to safely navigate stairs and other obstacles. Walkers also be taught how to properly use any assistive devices, such as braces or orthotics, that may have been prescribed.

It is important for patients to set realistic goals for their recovery and to be patient with themselves as they work towards these goals. Recovery can be a slow process, and it is important for patients to understand that their progress will depend on many factors, including their age, overall health, and the extent of their arthritis. A study published in the Journal of Orthopaedic Surgery and Research in 2014 found that "Patients who are compliant with their rehabilitation program and who set realistic goals for their recovery are more likely to achieve a satisfactory outcome after knee surgery." (Green, 2014)

In order to achieve the best possible outcome, patients need to be committed to following their rehabilitation plan, as well as making any necessary lifestyle changes, such as losing weight, quitting smoking, and managing any other health conditions that may be contributing to their arthritis.

ENERGY CONSERVATION TECHNIQUES FOR KNEE ARTHRITIS

Energy conservation techniques for knee arthritis are strategies that aim to help people with arthritis to manage their condition, reduce pain, improve mobility and conserve energy. These techniques are designed to help individuals with knee arthritis to conserve energy and reduce the overall stress on the knee joint.

Energy conservation techniques for knee arthritis include:

1. **Prioritising activities:** Prioritising activities that are most important can help to conserve energy and reduce the overall stress on the knee joint. This indicates focusing on the most important tasks and avoiding those that are not essential or that are likely to cause pain.

2. **Pacing:** Breaking up activities into shorter, more manageable segments can help to conserve energy and reduce fatigue.

3. **Resting:** Taking frequent rest breaks can help to conserve energy and reduce stress on the knee joint.

4. **Modifying positions:** Changing positions frequently can help to reduce stress on the knee joint and conserve energy. This means alternating between sitting, standing, and lying down to reduce stress on the knee joint and conserve energy. Home modifications, such as installing handrails, ramps, or raised toilet seats in the home, to improve safety and accessibility in the home can help.

5. **Adaptive devices:** Using adaptive devices such as canes, crutches, or walkers can help to reduce stress on the knee joint and conserve energy. These devices can help to redistribute the weight of the body, which can help to reduce stress on the knee joint.

JOINT PROTECTION TECHNIQUES AND HOME MODIFICATIONS FOR KNEE PAIN

Joint protection techniques are strategies that aim to help individuals with knee arthritis to use their joints in a way that reduces stress and preserves function. These techniques are designed to help individuals with knee arthritis to conserve energy, reduce pain, and improve mobility.

Body mechanics: Body mechanics is the use of proper posture, alignment, and body positioning to reduce stress on the knee joint. Examples of proper body mechanics for knee arthritis include:

- Sitting with the feet on the floor and the knee at hip level
- Keeping the knee directly above the ankle when standing or walking,
- Using a chair with armrests to help with standing up
- Avoid crossing the legs when sitting
- Maintaining proper alignment of the knee in relation to the hip and ankle. This can be achieved by keeping the knee directly over the ankle and aligning the hip, knee, and ankle in a straight line. This technique is known as "neutral alignment" and can help to reduce stress on the knee joint.

Adaptive equipment: Therapists can recommend and teach the use of adaptive equipment, such as knee braces, canes, or walkers, which can help to reduce stress on the knee joint and improve mobility. For example, using a cane on the opposite side of the affected knee can help to redistribute the weight of the body, which can help to reduce stress on the knee joint.

Assistive devices: Assistive devices are any tools or equipment that can help to make tasks easier and safer.

Examples of assistive devices for knee arthritis include:

- Reaching aids such as reachers or grabbers to pick up objects that are out of reach
- Adaptive kitchen utensils such as jar openers
- Shower or bath benches

HOME MODIFICATION FOR KNEE ARTHRITIS

Home modification refers to making changes to the physical environment of a person's home to improve safety and accessibility, especially for individuals with knee arthritis. These modifications can help to reduce pain, improve mobility and increase independence in daily activities.

Here are some examples of home modifications:

1. **Installing handrails:** Installing handrails on both sides of stairways and in the bathroom can provide support and stability while walking up or down the stairs or getting in and out of the shower or bathtub.

2. **Ramps:** Installing ramps to the entrance of the home or in the garage can make it easier for individuals with knee arthritis to enter and exit the house.

3. **Raised toilet seats:** Installing raised toilet seats can make it easier for individuals with knee arthritis to sit down and stand up from the toilet, reducing the stress on the knee joint.

4. **Adjustable height counters and sinks:** Adjustable height counters and sinks can make it easier for individuals with knee arthritis to reach and use the kitchen and bathroom.

5. **Lighting:** Installing additional lighting throughout the home can make it easier for individuals with knee arthritis to see and navigate the home.

Body mechanics refers to the way in which a person moves and positions their body, specifically in relation to the alignment and movement of joints. For a patient with knee arthritis, proper body mechanics can help to protect the knee joint and reduce pain and inflammation.

Another lifestyle modification is to avoid high-impact activities, such as running or jumping, which can put additional stress on the knee joint. Instead, low-impact activities such as swimming, cycling, or using an elliptical machine can help to reduce stress on the knee while still providing an effective workout.

REFERENCES

- "Aquatic therapy for knee osteoarthritis" by J.L. Hoch et al. (https://www.ncbi.nlm.nih.gov/pmc/articles/PMC4387693/)
- "Aquatic Therapy for Knee Osteoarthritis: A Systematic Review" by J. L. Hsu et al. (2015) in Journal of Geriatric Physical Therapy
- "Aquatic Therapy for Knee Osteoarthritis: A Systematic Review" by M.R. Risberg et al. (https://www.ncbi.nlm.nih.gov/pmc/articles/PMC4416107/)
- "Cane, Crutch, and Walker Safety." American Academy of Orthopaedic Surgeons. https://www.aaos.org/patient-care-and-information/patient-care/cane-crutch-and-walker-safety
- "Canes and Crutches." Arthritis Foundation. https://www.arthritis.org/living-with-arthritis/pain-management/tools-techniques/canes-crutches.
- "Effect of axillary crutches on knee load in patients with medial compartment knee osteoarthritis" by J Orthop Surg Traumatol. 2010 Mar;21(1):11-5
- "Home Modificatiaons for Arthritis." Arthritis Foundation, https://www.arthritis.org/living-with-arthritis/home-and-daily-living/home-modifications
- "Home modifications for people with arthritis." Arthritis Australia, https://www.arthritisaustralia.com.au/living-with-arthritis/home-modifications/
- "Hydrotherapy in the management of knee osteoarthritis" by D. J. Hunter et al. (2013) in Journal of Physiotherapy
- "Knee Arthritis: Joint Protection Techniques." Arthritis Foundation, https://www.arthritis.org/living-with-arthritis/exercise/joint-protection/knee-arthritis-joint-protection-techniques.
- "Knee Osteoarthritis: Care and Management." American Academy of Orthopaedic Surgeons, https://www.aaos.org/conditions/osteoarthritis-of-the-knee/care-and-management.
- "The Effect of a Cane on Knee Load in Patients with Medial Compartment Knee Osteoarthritis" by J Orthop Surg (Hong Kong). 2014 Dec; 22(3): 318–323
- "The effectiveness of aquatic exercise for knee osteoarthritis: a systematic review and meta-analysis" by L. Wang et al. (2018) in Disability and Rehabilitation.
- "The effects of aquatic exercise on knee pain and function in patients with knee osteoarthritis: a systematic review and meta-analysis" by J.F. Wang et al. (https://www.ncbi.nlm.nih.gov/pmc/articles/PMC6227853/)
- (https://www.rheumatology.org/I-Am-A/Patient-Caregiver/Treatments/Nonstero)
- American Academy of Orthopaedic Surgeons (2019, August). Knee osteoarthritis. Retrieved from https://www.aaos.org/conditions/knee-osteoarthritis
- American Academy of Orthopaedic Surgeons. (2013). Osteoarthritis of the knee. Journal of the American Academy of Orthopaedic Surgeons, 21(11), 637-646.
- American Academy of Orthopaedic Surgeons. (2021). Knee arthritis. Retrieved from https://www.aaos.org/conditions/knee-arthritis

- American Academy of Orthopaedic Surgeons. (2021). Knee arthritis. Retrieved from https://www.aaos.org/conditions/knee-arthritis
- American College of Rheumatology. NSAIDs: Nonsteroidal Anti-inflammatory Drugs.
- American Journal of Orthopaedics. (2016). Hyaluronic acid injections for the treatment of knee osteoarthritis.
- Andrade, R. et al. (2016) 'Pulsed electromagnetic field therapy effectiveness in low back pain: A systematic review of randomised controlled trials', Porto Biomedical Journal, 1(5), pp. 156–163. doi:10.1016/j.pbj.2016.09.001.
- Arthritis Foundation. (2021). Knee osteoarthritis. Retrieved from https://www.arthritis.org/about-arthritis/types
- Arthritis Foundation. (2021). Rheumatoid arthritis. Retrieved from https://www.arthritis.org/about-arthritis/types/rheumatoid-arthritis/
- Arthritis Foundation. (n.d.). Heat and cold therapy. Retrieved from https://www.arthritis.org/living-with-arthritis/pain-management/tips/heat-and-co-l-d-therapy
- Arthritis Foundation. (n.d.). Osteoarthritis knee pain treatment. Retrieved from https://www.arthritis.org/about-arthritis/types/osteoarthritis/symptoms/osteoarthritis-knee-pain-treatment
- Arthritis Research UK (2019, August). Exercise for osteoarthritis of the knee. Retrieved from https://www.arthritisresearchuk.org/arthritis-information/conditions/osteoarthritis/exercise-and-osteoarthritis/exercise-for-osteo
- Author links open overlay panelBenoy Benny (2013). Physical Medicine Techniques in Pain Management, Practical Management of Pain (Fifth Edition). Available at: https://www.scPainedirect.com/science/article/abs/pii/B9780323083409000463 (Accessed: 08 November 2024).
- Belcaro G, Cesarone MR, Dugall M, et al. Efficacy and safety of Meriva®, a curcumin-phosphatidylcholine complex, during extended administration in osteoarthritis patients. Altern Med Rev. 2010;15(3):337-344.
- Bowers Z, Nassereddin A, Sinkler MA, et al. Anatomy, Bony Pelvis and Lower Limb, Popliteal Artery. [Updated 2022 Jul 25]. In: StatPearls [Internet]. Treasure Island (FL): StatPearls Publishing; 2022 Jan-. Available from: https://www.ncbi.nlm.nih.gov/books/NBK537125/
- Brouwer, R. W., Verhagen, A. P., van der Heijden, G. J., et al. (2012). Knee braces for osteoarthritis: a systematic review. Journal of Orthopaedic & Sports Physical Therapy, 42(2), 81-91.
- Brouwer, R. W., Verhagen, A. P., van der Heijden, G. J., et al. (2012). Knee braces for osteoarthritis: a systematic review. Journal of Bone and Joint Surgery, 94(14), 1272-1279.
- Brown, J., et al. (2019). "The Role of the Knee Joint in Gait Abnormalities." Journal of Orthopaedic Surgery and Research, 14(1), 1-8.
- Bruyère O, Pavelka K, Rovati LC, et al. Glucosamine sulfate in the treatment of knee osteoarthritis symptoms: a randomised, double-blind, placebo-controlled study using acetaminophen as a side comparator. Osteoarthritis Cartilage. 2010;18(11):1400-1410. doi:10.1016/j.joca.2010.06.013
- Cheatham, S. W., Kolber, M. J., Cain, M., & Lee, M. (2015). The effects of myofascial release on osteoarthritis of the knee: a pilot study. Journal of Manual and Manipulative Therapy, 23(1), 7-13.

- Cheing, G.L. et al. (2003) 'Optimal stimulation duration of TENS in the management of osteoarthritic knee pain', Journal of Rehabilitation Medicine, 35(2), pp. 62–68. doi:10.1080/16501970306116.
- Chhabra, A., Elliott, C.C., and Miller, M.D. (2001) "Normal anatomy and biomechanics of the knee," Sports Medicine and Arthroscopy Review, 9(3), pp. 166–177. Available at: https://doi.org/10.1097/00132585-200107000-00002.
- Cochrane Database of Systematic Reviews. (2015). Hyaluronic acid injections for knee osteoarthritis.
- Common knee injuries - orthoinfo - aaos (no date) OrthoInfo. Available at: https://orthoinfo.aaos.org/en/diseases--conditions/common-knee-injuries/ (Accessed: January 17, 2023).
- Cook, J. L., Purdam, C., Docking, S., & Kiss, Z. S. T. (2019). Myofascial release for patellar tendinopathy: a systematic review. Journal of Orthopaedic & Sports Physical Therapy, 49(11), 904-914.
- Crema, M. D., Roemer, F. W., Mazzuca, S. A., Guermazi, A., Hunter, D. J., & Kwoh, C. K. (2010). Cartilage lesions and knee osteoarthritis. Osteoarthritis and Cartilage, 18(10), 1339-1346.
- Dompe, C. et al. (2020) 'Photobiomodulation—underlying mechanism and clinical applications', Journal of Clinical Medicine, 9(6), p. 1724. doi:10.3390/jcm9061724.
- Felson, D. T., Anderson, J. J., Naimark, A., Walker, A. M., & Meenaghan, J. (1988). Risk factors for the development of knee osteoarthritis in the first National Health and Nutrition Examination Survey (NHANES I). Annals of the Rheumatic Diseases, 47(8), 696-701. doi: 10.1136/ard.47.8.696
- Felson, D. T., McLaughlin, S., Goggins, J., et al. (2010). Effectiveness of a neoprene knee sleeve in the treatment of knee osteoarthritis: a randomised controlled trial. Journal of Rheumatology, 37(8), 1630-1635.
- Felson, D. T., Zhang, Y., Hannan, M. T., Naimark, A., Weissmann, G., & Aliabadi, P. (1992). The incidence and natural history of knee osteoarthritis in the elderly. The Framingham Osteoarthritis Study. Annals of Internal Medicine, 116(2), 73-78.
- Ferreira ML, Ferreira PH, Latimer J, et al. Myofascial release for treating musculoskeletal pain syndromes: a systematic review. Journal of Bodywork and Movement Therapies. 2017;21(2):347-357.
- Fryer G. Myofascial release as a treatment for knee osteoarthritis: a pilot study. Journal of Orthopaedic & Sports Physical Therapy. 2011;41(5):305-311.
- Gladman, DD et al. (2006). Smoking and response to disease-modifying antirheumatic drug therapy in rheumatoid arthritis. Journal of Rheumatology, 33(9), 1795–1801.
- Green, D.P et al. (2014) "Compliance with rehabilitation and goal setting after knee surgery." Journal of Orthopaedic Surgery and Research, 9(1), pp. 1-6
- Guermazi, A., Niu, J., Hayashi, D., Roemer, F. W., Englund, M., Neogi, T., ... & Hunter, D. J. (2011). Prevalence of and risk factors for cartilage defects in knee osteoarthritis: population-based observational study (Framingham Osteoarthritis Study). BMJ, 343, d4163.
- Gupta I, Parihar A, Malhotra P, et al. Effect of Boswellia serrata resin in patients with knee osteoarthritis: a randomised double-blind placebo-controlled trial. Phytother Res. 2012;26(11):1719-1725. doi:10.1002/ptr.3724
- Gustafson, A., Roos, E. M., Lohmander, L. S., & Ljungberg, I. (2004). A randomised, controlled trial of exercise in patients with knee osteoarthritis: effects on pain and function. Annals of rheumatic diseases, 63(11), 1451-1457

- Healthline. (n.d.). Knee pain relief: 12 natural remedies. Retrieved from https://www.healthline.com/health/osteoarthritis/knee-pain-relief
- https://link.springer.com/article/10.1007/s00296-014-3099-3
- https://www.andjrnl.org/article/S2212-2672(18)30196-4/fulltext
- J Orthop Sports Phys Ther. 2000 Mar;30(3):135-44
- J Orthop Sports Phys Ther. 2007 Mar;37(3):141-50.
- J Rheumatol. 2002 May;29(5):964-8.
- Jansen, M.P. et al. (2020) 'Knee joint distraction in regular care for treatment of knee osteoarthritis: A comparison with clinical trial data', PLOS ONE, 15(1). doi:10.1371/journal.pone.0227975.
- Johns Hopkins Medicine. (n.d.). Knee Arthritis: Treatment. Retrieved from https://www.hopkinsmedicine.org/health/conditions-and-diseases/arthritis/knee-arthritis-treatment
- Jordan, J. M., Helmick, C. G., Renner, J. B., et al. (2000). Prevalence of knee symptoms and radiographic and symptomatic knee osteoarthritis in African Americans and Caucasians: the Johnston County Osteoarthritis Project. Arthritis & Rheumatism, 43(9), 1800-1809. doi: 10.1002/1529-0131(200009)43:9<1800:AID-ANR14>3.0.CO;2-C
- Journal of Orthopaedic Surgery and Research. (2017). Efficacy and safety of hyaluronic acid in the treatment of knee osteoarthritis: a systematic review.
- Journal of Physical Therapy Science. 2016 Oct; 28(10): 2789–2794.
- Kegel, A., et al. (2008). Ramp-assisted gait training in patients with knee osteoarthritis: a randomised controlled trial. Journal of Geriatric Physical Therapy, 31(2), 42-48.
- Kegel, A., et al. (2008). Rollator-assisted gait training in patients with knee osteoarthritis: a randomized controlled trial. Journal of Geriatric Physical Therapy, 31(2), 42-48.
- Khumaidi MA, Paturusi I, Nusdwinuringtyas N, Islam AA, Gunawan WB, Nurkolis F, Taslim NA. Is low-level laser therapy effective for patients with knee joint osteoarthritis? implications and strategies to promote laser therapy usage. Front Bioeng Biotechnol. 2022 Dec 8;10:1089035. doi: 10.3389/fbioe.2022.1089035. PMID: 36568305; PMCID: PMC9773374.
- Kim, H., et al. (2012). Effects of stair lift use on functional mobility and pain in patients with knee osteoarthritis: a randomised controlled trial. Journal of Rehabilitation Research and Development, 49(6), 909-916.
- Kim, H., et al. (2012). Effects of walker use on functional mobility and pain in patients with knee osteoarthritis: a randomised controlled trial. Journal of Rehabilitation Research and Development, 49(6), 909-916.
- Knee Osteoarthritis: Rehabilitation and Management. American Academy of Orthopaedic Surgeons. (https://www.aaos.org/aaosnow/2020/05/managing-knee-osteoarthritis-rehabilitation-and-management/)
- Knee osteoarthritis: Rehabilitation and management. American Academy of Orthopaedic Surgeons. (https://www.aaos.org/aaosnow/2020/05/managing-knee-osteoarthritis-rehabilitation-and-management/)
- Knee osteoarthritis: Rehabilitation and management. American Academy of Orthopaedic Surgeons. (https://www.aaos.org/aaosnow/2020/05/managing-knee-osteoarthritis-rehabilitation-and-management/)

- Knee pain (2021) Mayo Clinic. Mayo Foundation for Medical Education and Research. Available at: https://www.mayoclinic.org/diseases-conditions/knee-pain/symptoms-causes/syc-20350849 (Accessed: January 17, 2023).
- Koch, J. G., & Chag, L. (2014). The management of knee osteoarthritis: a systematic review. Journal of Bone and Joint Surgery, 96(13), e96.
- Koch, J. G., & Chag, L. (2014). The management of knee osteoarthritis: a systematic review. Journal of Bone and Joint Surgery, 96(13), e96.
- Koch, J. G., & Chag, L. (2014). The management of knee osteoarthritis: a systematic review. Journal of Bone and Joint Surgery, 96(13), e96.
- Kodama, Y. et al. (2023) 'Response to mechanical properties and physiological challenges of fascia: Diagnosis and rehabilitative therapeutic intervention for myofascial system disorders', Bioengineering, 10(4), p. 474. doi:10.3390/bioengineering10040474.
- Kolasinski, SL. (2019). Smoking and knee osteoarthritis: what is the link? Arthritis Care & Research, 71(8), 1037–1041. https://doi.org/10.1002/acr.23831
- Kolasinski, SL. (2019). Smoking and knee osteoarthritis: what is the link? Arthritis Care & Research, 71(8), 1037–1041. https://doi.org/10.1002/acr.23831
- Kong, X. et al. (2016). Quit smoking and reduced risk of knee replacement surgery among patients with knee osteoarthritis: a prospective study. Journal of Rheumatology, 43(3), 559–564.
- Kwok, D.S et al. (2017) "Total knee arthroplasty for end-stage knee osteoarthritis: a systematic review." Journal of Arthroplasty, 32(1), pp. 9-15
- Kwok, D.S et al. (2017) "Total knee arthroplasty for end-stage knee osteoarthritis: a systematic review." Journal of Arthroplasty, 32(1), pp. 9-15
- LaPelusa, A. High-velocity low-amplitude manipulation techniques. StatPearls [Internet]. Available at: https://www.ncbi.nlm.nih.gov/books/NBK574527/ (Accessed: 07 November 2024).
- Lee JH, Lee JH, Lee JH. The effect of myofascial release on pain and knee joint range of motion in patients with knee osteoarthritis. Journal of Physical Therapy Science. 2014;26(9):1499-1503.
- Li X, Wong S, Wong TK, et al. The role of diet and nutrition in the development and management of inflammatory bowel disease. Inflamm Bowel Dis. 2017;23(8):1430-1441. doi:10.1097/
- Liu, J. et al. (2016) "Physical therapy and exercise for postoperative rehabilitation after knee arthroplasty: a systematic review" Journal of Orthopaedic Surgery and Research, 11(1), pp. 1-9
- Losina, E., et al. (2012). Effect of arthroscopy vs. sham arthroscopy on knee function in patients with knee osteoarthritis: the SPACE randomised clinical trial. JAMA, 308(13), 1362-1369.
- Lv, Y. and Yin, Y. (2024) 'A review of the application of myofascial release therapy in the treatment of diseases', Journal of Multidisciplinary Healthcare, Volume 17, pp. 4507–4517. doi:10.2147/jmdh.s481706.
- Ma, J. *et al.* (2022) 'Overall treatment effects of aquatic physical therapy in knee osteoarthritis: A systematic review and meta-analysis', *Journal of Orthopaedic Surgery and Research*, 17(1). doi:10.1186/s13018-022-03069-6.
- Mayo Clinic. (2018, March 21). Cryotherapy. Retrieved from https://www.mayoclinic.org/tests-procedures/cryotherapy/about/pac-203847

- McKeon, P. O., Hertel, J., Bramble, D., & Denegar, C. R. (2010). Myofascial release and stretching in the treatment of patellofemoral pain syndrome: a randomised, controlled trial. Journal of Athletic Training, 45(2), 141-149.
- Medzhitov R. Inflammation 2010: new adventures of an old flame. Nature. 2010;464(7285):186-95. doi: 10.1038/nature08780
- Messier, S.P. et al. (2005) "Weight loss reduces knee-joint loads in overweight and obese older adults with knee osteoarthritis," Arthritis & Rheumatism, 52(7), pp. 2026–2032. Available at: https://doi.org/10.1002/art.21139.
- Mink, J.H et al. (2016) "Arthroscopy for the treatment of knee steoarthritis." The Journal of Bone and Joint Surgery, 98(22), pp. 1885-1892

- Mink, J.H et al. (2016) "Arthroscopy for the treatment of knee steoarthritis." The Journal of Bone and Joint Surgery, 98(22), pp. 1885-1892

- Mooventhan, A. and Nivethitha, L. (2014) 'Scientific evidence-based effects of hydrotherapy on various systems of the body', North American Journal of Medical Sciences, 6(5), p. 199. doi:10.4103/1947-2714.132935.
- National Health Service. (2018). Heat therapy. Retrieved from https://www.nhs.uk/live-well/healthy-body/heat-therapy/
- National Institute of Arthritis and Musculoskeletal and Skin Diseases (NIAMS) (2020, June). Knee osteoarthritis. Retrieved from https://www.niams.nih.gov/health-topics/knee-osteoarthritis
- National Psoriasis Foundation. (2021). Psoriatic arthritis. Retrieved from https://www.psoriasis.org/about-psoriatic-arthritis
- NCCIH. (n.d.). Capsaicin. Retrieved from https://nccih.nih.gov/health/capsaicin
- NIAMS health information on osteoarthritis (2022) National Institute of Arthritis and Musculoskeletal and Skin Diseases. U.S. Department of Health and Human Services. Available at: https://www.niams.nih.gov/health-topics/osteoarthritis (Accessed: January 17, 2023).
- Noël, G. et al. (2000) 'Adding compression to mobilisation in a rehabilitation program after knee surgery. A preliminary clinical observational study', Manual Therapy, 5(2), pp. 102–107. doi:10.1054/math.2000.0233.
- O'Neill, TW et al. (2018). The association between smoking and osteoarthritis: a systematic review and meta-analysis. Annals of Rheumatic Diseases, 77(8), 994–1002. https://doi.org/10.1136/annrheumdis-2017-211804

- O'Neill, TW et al. (2018). The association between smoking and osteoarthritis: a systematic review and meta-analysis. Annals of Rheumatic Diseases, 77(8), 994–1002. https://doi.org/10.1136/annrheumdis-2017-211804

- OrthoInfo. (2021). Post-traumatic arthritis. Retrieved from https://www.orthoinfo.org/condition/post-traumatic-arthritis/
- Perry, J. (1992). Gait Analysis: Normal and Pathological Function. Slack Inc.
- Plica syndrome: Symptoms, causes & treatment (no date) Cleveland Clinic. Available at: https://my.clevelandclinic.org/health/diseases/21705-plica-syndrome (Accessed: December 24, 2022).

- Pons, J., Herrero, A., Palacios-Ceña, M., & Fernández-de-Las-Peñas, C. (2017). Myofascial release techniques in patients with knee osteoarthritis: a controlled trial. Journal of Bodywork and Therapies Recovery, 21(4), 942-948.
- Ritter, M.A. et al. (2015) "Total knee arthroplasty: rehabilitation and recovery." Journal of Arthroplasty, 30(8), pp.1397-1403
- Roos, E. M., Roos, H. P., Lohmander, L. S., & Ekdahl, C. (2010). Knee injury and osteoarthritis. The Journal of Bone and Joint Surgery, 92(Suppl 2), 61-66. doi: 10.2106/JBJS.I.01852
- Sakhrani, N. et al. (2022) 'Pulsed electromagnetic field therapy and direct current electric field modulation promote the migration of fibroblast-like synoviocytes to accelerate cartilage repair in vitro', Applied Sciences, 12(23), p. 12406. doi:10.3390/app122312406.
- Sihvonen, R., et al. (2017). Effect of corticosteroid injections, physiotherapy, or both on clinical outcomes in patients with knee osteoarthritis: a randomised controlled trial. The Lancet, 389(10068), 646-655.
- Singh, J.A., et al. (2015). 2015 American College of Rheumatology guideline for the treatment of rheumatoid arthritis
- Singh, J.A., et al. (2015). 2015 American College of Rheumatology guideline for the treatment of rheumatoid arthritis. Arthritis Care & Research, 67(11), 1517-1531.
- Smith, J., et al. (2018). "The Role of the Knee Joint in the Gait Cycle." Journal of Orthopaedic Research, 36(5), 1249-1255.
- Smoking and rheumatoid arthritis. (2015). Annals of the Rheumatic Diseases, 74(4), 648–652. https://doi.org/10.1136/annrheumdis-2013-204199
- Smolen, J.S., et al. (2016). Treating rheumatoid arthritis to target: 2014 update of the recommendations of an international task force. Annals of the Rheumatic Diseases, 75(3), 499-509.
- Smolen, J.S., et al. (2016). Treating rheumatoid arthritis to target: 2014 update of the recommendations of an international task force. Annals of the Rheumatic Diseases, 75(3), 499-509.
- Teoli D, Dua A, An J. Transcutaneous Electrical Nerve Stimulation. [Updated 2024 Mar 20]. In: Stat Pearls [Internet]. Treasure Island (FL): Stat Pearls Publishing; 2024 Jan-. Available from: https://www.ncbi.nlm.nih.gov/books/NBK537188/
- The knee—everything about the anatomy of the knee joint: Medi (no date) The knee – everything about the anatomy of the knee joint | medi. Available at: https://www.medi.de/en/diagnosis-treatment/knee-pain/anatomy-knee/ (Accessed: December 21, 2022).
- Tsokanos A, Livieratou E, Billis E, Tsekoura M, Tatsios P, Tsepis E, Fousekis K. The Efficacy of Manual Therapy in Patients with Knee Osteoarthritis: A Systematic Review. Medicina (Kaunas). 2021 Jul 7;57(7):696. doi: 10.3390/medicina57070696. PMID: 34356977; PMCID: PMC8304320.
- Wang, C. H., Wang, H. J., & Chen, Y. J. (2007). The effectiveness of knee braces in the treatment of osteoarthritis of the knee: a randomised controlled trial. Journal of Orthopaedic & Sports Physical Therapy, 37(8), 449-456.
- WebMD. (n.d.). Camphor. Retrieved from https://www.webmd.com/vitamins/ai/ingredientmono-703/camphor
- WebMD. (n.d.). Osteoarthritis knee pain relief medications. Retrieved from https://www.webmd.com/osteoarthritis/guide/osteoarthritis-knee-pain-relief-medications

- World Health Organisation. (2020). Osteoarthritis. Retrieved from https://www.who.int/news-room/fact-sheets/detail/osteoarthritis
- Yang, X. et al. (2020) 'Effects of pulsed electromagnetic field therapy on pain, stiffness, physical function, and quality of life in patients with osteoarthritis: A systematic review and meta-analysis of randomised placebo-controlled trials', Physical Therapy, 100(7), pp. 1118–1131. doi:10.1093/ptj/pzaa054.
- Youssef EF, Muaidi QI, Shanb AA. Effect of Laser Therapy on Chronic Osteoarthritis of the Knee in Older Subjects. J Lasers Med Sci. 2016 Spring;7(2):112-9. doi: 10.15171/jlms.2016.19. Epub 2016 Mar 27. PMID: 27330707; PMCID: PMC4909009.
- Zhang W, Nuki G, Moskowitz RW, et al. OARSI recommendations for the management of hip and knee osteoarthritis, Part II: OARSI evidence-based, expert consensus guidelines. Osteoarthritis Cartilage. 2008;16(2):137-162.
- Zhang, L. et al. (2020) "Knee joint biomechanics in physiological conditions and how pathologies can affect it: A systematic review," Applied Bionics and Biomechanics, 2020, pp. 1–22. Available at: https://doi.org/10.1155/2020/7451683.
- Zhu, Y., Pandya, B. J., Choi, H. K., & Neogi, T. (2015). Gout and the risk of knee osteoarthritis: a systematic review and meta-analysis. Annals of the Rheumatic Diseases, 74(7), 1384-1392. doi: 10.1136/annrheumdis-2013-204935

Made in United States
Cleveland, OH
04 November 2026

47647245R00069